# Family Home Care:

## Critical Issues for Services and Policies

Robert Perlman, PhD, is a teacher and researcher in the field of social welfare and has written on policy issues in the social services. He has practiced as a social worker and as a social planner in the 1960s. Since 1965, he has been a member of the faculty of the Florence Heller Graduate School at Brandeis University, Waltham, Massachusetts. He is author of *Consumers and Social Services* (Wiley, 1975) and coauthor of *Community Organization and Social Planning* (Wiley and Council on Social Work Education, 1972) and of *Families in the Energy Crisis* (Ballinger, 1977).

# Family Home Care:
## Critical Issues for Services and Policies

Robert Perlman, PhD
Editor

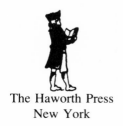

The Haworth Press
New York

*Family Home Care: Critical Issues for Services and Policies* has also been published as *Home Health Care Services Quarterly*, Volume 3, Numbers 3/4, Fall/Winter 1982.

The Haworth Press, Inc., 28 East 22 Street, New York, NY 10010

**Library of Congress Cataloging in Publication Data**
Main entry under title:

Family home care.

"Has also been published as Home health care services quarterly, volume 3, number 3/4, fall/winter 1982"—P.
Includes bibliographies.
1. Handicapped—Home care—United States—Addresses, essays, lectures. 2. Handicapped—Government policy—United States—Addresses, essays, lectures. I. Perlman, Robert.
HV1553.F35      1983            362.8'28'0973            83-81
ISBN 0-86656-220-6
ISBN 0-86656-221-4 (soft)

To Pink

# Family Home Care:
## Critical Issues for Services and Policies

Home Health Care Services Quarterly
Volume 3, Numbers 3/4

## CONTENTS

*The Introductory Sections were written by the editor. References used in these sections appear at the end of the book.*

MONNICA C. STEWART, MB, BS, D(Obst), RCOG, *Community Medicine Physician, City and East London Area Health Authority, London, United Kingdom*

ANN-MARIE THOM, *Executive Director, Visiting Nurse Association of New York, New York, New York*

PATRICIA THOMAS, *Executive Director, Visiting Homemakers Association, Toronto, Ontario, Canada*

THOMAS R. WILLEMAIN, PhD, *Associate Professor of Public Policy, John F. Kennedy School of Government, Harvard University, Cambridge, Massachusetts; Senior Research Associate, University Health Policy Consortium, Brandeis University, Waltham, Massachusetts*

JUDITH LA VOR WILLIAMS, *Florence Heller School for Advanced Studies in Social Welfare, Brandeis University, Waltham, Massachusetts*

# Editorial

The role of the family in modern life is being considered with intense interest because of demographic changes in the populations of the western world. The family has been the subject of myth, idealization, mistrust with respect to the forces of goodwill found in family relationships and unrealistic expectation.

In *Family Home Care* a group of knowledgeable authors present the family in all of its aspects: as a practical resource, as a less tangible but nonetheless important support, as an institution affected by substantial changes in physical and economic circumstances. Implicit in the presentation is recognition of the need for coherent family policy based upon the realities of the modern world.

The editors of *Home Health Care Services Quarterly* are pleased to present *Family Home Care* as a contribution to the literature of this important subject.

*B.T.*
*L.R.*

# Foreword

Professor Perlman has gathered together an unusual and useful set of papers dealing with family home care. It is an unusual set because it includes the views not only of practitioners in the field of family home care, but also professors of history, sociology, and public health. It focuses not only on the elderly, but also handicapped children and young people. It is not often that such a range of perspectives is presented in a single volume. The papers are useful in that they are at the cutting edge of the conventional wisdom regarding family home care—a topic that has taken on renewed interest with the advent of the Reagan administration. In a few places, there are signs that we may be moving beyond the conventional wisdom and toward a better understanding of the real issues involved in family home care. The book is also particularly useful because of Professor Perlman's own analytic contribution at the beginning of each of the sections. There he gives a preview of the articles to follow, and fits their themes into the context of the major issues being considered. This is a fine service for the readers and prepares them for the articles coming up; but also introduces additional material not found in any of the articles. Such a contribution on Professor Perlman's part, however, reduces the number of things that one can say in a Preface because he has already said them so well. I would not want, therefore, to repeat what you will read in the following pages but, rather, take this opportunity to grind a few axes of my own.

First, I would ask the reader not to miss the excellent material in the article by Professors Perlman and Giele, entitled "An Unstable Triad: Dependents' Demands, Family Resources, Community Supports." While much of the information presented there has been presented elsewhere, they offer some new and original material which has not yet been published. This material deals with their analysis of the 1976 *Survey of Income and Education* to arrive at an estimate of the dependent population, their needs, and their care arrangements. Using this large data base, they attempt to measure the "burden" that a dependent member places on the family. They do this by creating an index of family time potential, constructing it from separate items in the survey. Time has been identified as one of the key indicators of stress and strain on caretakers, and the Perlman-Giele approach offers an opportunity to get some idea of the national magnitude of the caring endeavor.

Farber's article, "Sociological Ambivalence and the Family," presents the concept "normality of disapppointment" as it applies to retarded children. This idea can be extended to the elderly and provides a useful counterweight to what I believe is a growing mind set that denies the losses that accompany old age. While it is certainly true that older people can be productive, creative, intellectually stimulating, contributors to society, and all the rest, there is in fact a set of losses that accompanies aging into the seventies and the eighties. These include: loss of role, loss of jobs, loss of certain functions, loss of spouse and, ultimately, loss of one's own life. The current mood, and the interest in creating more and more services for the elderly, denies these losses and/or assumes that they can be compensated for by professionally or non-professionally provided services. Farber's notion of "the normality of disappointment" is an important consideration. It brings into focus the issue of just how far into the store of human misery public responsibility should extend. Is there some irreducible level of pain and suffering that cannot be compensated for by our public or private interventions, and which each of us as individuals or families must bear?

Robert Moroney has been one of the clearest thinkers on the role of families and public policy, and he talks about the shared responsibility between the two groups. His notion, held by many others, that families are service providers is one that has disturbed me for a long time. This concept takes a set of reciprocal inter-actions within a primary group and then conceptualizes them in the service-giving model taken from the professional sector. This approach defines certain behavior as services being provided by family members to their dependent elders or adults. Preparing a meal becomes a food service; cleaning the house becomes a home-maker service; emptying a bedpan becomes a personal care service; going out to do the shopping becomes a transportation service. The dependent individual then becomes a costly user of these services, whether they are priced in terms of the usual wages in the com-munity or of opportunity costs. What gets lost in this equation is the kind of contribution that the "dependent" person makes to that primary group. The older woman who requires shopping assistance has just finished knitting a prom dress for her grand-daughter; the dependent aunt for whom the bedpan has been emptied has for years been the "significant other" for her retarded niece (a psychiatric service?); the wheelchair-bound father-in-law has just called in some of his chips and made arrrangements with the local banker and lawyer to set up his son-in-law in business. The service equation looks only at the costs of what is provided the older person; it does not take into account the contributions that are made by other members of a primary group on a reciprocal basis. It will be very important to get out of this trap, otherwise dependent people will be further devalued on one hand, and become too expensive on the other.

An increasingly important area for exploration is that of self-help and self-care. This movement will expand in the future, not only because of the way social interactions have been "cashed out," but also because it brings with it more autonomy and control to the person involved. The interest in family care is sparked not only by the cost, but also by the fact that it is becoming new territory into which professionals can move. Dying now has become the territory for a host of professionals who enter under the umbrella of "hospice." Somehow, the people will have to pull back to themselves the responsibility for care and decision-making.

It seems to me that the key problem in family care, particularly of the elderly, is "how do we maintain the dignity and worth of older persons in the face of real losses and dependencies?" Older persons are not a class or a group to which we can relate objectively. It is easy to be objective about blacks or Chinese or children for, unless we are in one of these groups already, we will never become a member. Each of us, however, will definitely join the elderly group (none of us assumes that he or she will be dead). Attitudes toward older persons swing between denial of growing dependency on one hand, to overprotection on the other. As we develop more and more ways of helping the elderly, it becomes more necessary to develop a philosophy and an approach that maximizes a person's autonomy and decision-making in a situation of increasing dependence on others. This is a public policy issue which impacts on individuals—you and me. I hope that we will handle it correctly, because I am not getting any younger either.

Professor Perlman's book, *Family Home Care* will cause all of us to think more deeply about these important issues.

*James J. Callahan, Jr., PhD*
*Director, Levinson Policy Institute*
*Heller School, Brandeis University*
*September 8, 1982*

# List of Contributors

**Francis G. Caro**, Director of the Institute for Social Welfare Research at the Community Service Society of New York

**Gerben DeJong**, Senior Research Associate and Assistant Professor, Department of Rehabilitation Medicine, Tufts-New England Medical Center, Boston

**John Demos**, Professor of History, Brandeis University

**Bernard Farber**, Professor of Sociology, Arizona State University, Tempe

**Dwight L. Frankfather**, Assistant Professor, University of Chicago School of Social Service Administration

**Janet Z. Giele**, Associate Professor, The Heller School, Brandeis University

**Aileen Florita Hart**, Associate Professor, Chairperson, Social Policy Sequence, Simmons College School of Social Work

**Charles R. Horejsi**, Professor of Social Work, University of Montana

**Lorraine V. Klerman**, Professor of Public Health, The Heller School, Brandeis University

**Abraham Monk**, Brookdale Professor of Gerontology, School of Social Work, Columbia University

**Bonnie Brown Morell**, Planner, Division of Mental Health, Mental Retardation and Substance Abuse Services, Raleigh, North Carolina

**Robert M. Moroney**, Professor of Social Policy and Planning, School of Social Work, Arizona State University, Tempe

**Robert Morris**, Emeritus Professor, The Heller School, Brandeis University

**Alan Sager**, Assistant Professor of Urban and Health Planning, The Heller School, Brandeis University

**Steven P. Segal**, Professor, School of Social Welfare, University of California, Berkeley

**Michael J. Smith**, Assistant Professor, Hunter College School of Social Work

# Acknowledgments

Three of the papers in this collection were prepared for a conference jointly sponsored by the Massachusetts Foundation for Humanities and Public Policy, a program of the National Endowment for the Humanities, and the Florence Heller Graduate School for Advanced Studies in Social Welfare of Brandeis University. The papers were presented by John Demos, Robert Moroney, and Robert Morris at the conference in 1978.

I am indebted to Professor Mary Ann Glendon of the Boston College Law School and to Professor Saul Touster of Brandeis University for their assistance in exploring the legal aspects of this subject.

The paper by Janet Zollinger Giele and myself was developed for a workshop on family care, in connection with a training program concerned with public policy and the family funded by the Center for Studies of Metropolitan Problems of the National Institute of Mental Health.

I want to express my appreciation to Rosemary and Gunnar Dybwad and to Sylvia Pendleton for their help in locating written materials in an emerging field of inquiry and to Ruth Daniels for her patient, painstaking work in preparing the manuscript.

*Robert Perlman*
*Brandeis University*
*August 1982*

# PART I: OVERVIEW

# Introduction to Part I

Each year more and more disabled and dependent people must look to someone else for help with the simple yet crucial things that most of us do for ourselves—washing and dressing, eating, toileting, getting to work and school, household chores, and shopping. Upwards of four million people living at home receive this kind of personal care from their parents, spouses, or children. American families provide three times as much of this vital caring as all the nursing homes, hospitals, and institutions combined.

But this large system of family care is fragile and unstable. Urgent problems have emerged for all concerned.

The numbers of dependent people of all ages and the severity of their disabilities are steadily increasing, primarily as a result of developments in health care. At one end of the spectrum are the survivors of birth defects. At the other end are the frail elderly now living in substantial numbers into their 90s and 100s. As the degree of their impairment grows, so do the demands they must make on their families' time, energy, finances, emotional commitment, and other resources.

At the same time the ability and willingness of families to meet demands that can become heavy may be diminishing as a result of changes in family size and composition, shifts in employment patterns and sex-related roles, and in people's ideas of what is morally right, socially accepted, and personally desirable.

The growth in the dependent population and the changes in family behavior now pose mounting problems for social policies and programs in this and other industrialized countries. The main alternative to family home care is institutional care, the cost of

*1*

which has been rising precipitously on an individual basis and as a total social expenditure. Even a small diminution in the effort of families would confront legislators, taxpayers, and providers of institutional care with staggering financial and administrative burdens. On the other hand, expanding public services to assist families to provide care at home raises profound questions about the proper spheres of individual, family, and public responsibility at a time when the Welfare State in general is under attack.

This book is about these issues in family home care, by which we mean the provision of personal, non-professional services and support by one or more members of a family to someone who is dependent as a result of physical, mental, or emotional impairment or disability. This definition excludes certain situations, such as that of the single-person household. We are dealing with arrangements in which the dependent person shares the same residence with his or her family. Generally this around-the-clock responsibility is more intensive and demanding than taking care of a disabled relative who lives nearby. Nor does our focus include a significant and increasing number of people who either have no family ties or such tenuous ones that they cannot expect assistance from relatives.

Our subject is part of the larger problem of long-term care of the disabled, but the focus here is on *care given in the home by family members*. Though professional and paraprofessional services may also be provided, the emphasis is on the responsibility taken by the family for daily care without which the dependent person could not remain out of an institution. Home care entails a continuing commitment by the family to an arrangement that persists for months and often for years.

Two perspectives are stressed in this book. One is the emphasis on the family and the other is the inclusion of a wide range of ages and disabilities. Both the organization of services and the research literature tend to give more prominence to the individuals at risk than to the families involved in home care. This has been called the "concentric approach," which places the problems, needs, and feelings of the dependent person at the core of the situation (Kew, 1975). The life of the family, Kew argues, should be the point of departure in setting policy and organizing services.

The disadvantages of the concentric approach were pointed out in a study of social services to handicapped children and their families which concluded that in general, services received by handicapped children and their families tend to be child-oriented rather than family-oriented, (a pattern) clearly at odds with the demonstrated effectiveness of family-oriented services in preventing out-of-home placements and with the national social policy initiatives to promote the abilities of families to care for their handicapped children in their own homes (Krauss and MacEachron, 1981).

Our definition of family home care encompasses a broad spectrum of individuals who, though they differ in age, the nature of their disability or dependency, and the characteristics of their families, nonetheless have much in common. We speak here of the mentally retarded, the physically handicapped, the incapacitated mental patient, and the largest and fastest growing group, the frail elderly, all of whom share an inability to function independently. It is remarkable to what extent the circumstances and problems of these apparently disparate populations are similar.

Clearly there are important differences in the needs of a three-year-old retarded child with multiple disabilities and an 80-year-old bedfast woman. It is our contention, however, that from the perspectives of the individuals involved, the families, and the public, the similarities outweigh the differences. Our concern is with the element of *dependency* and not with the specific nature of the disability, impairment, loss of function, or handicap. There are many people who are able to function independently or with a bare minimum of help—some of them living alone—who have serious physical deficits and disabilities. What is critical in this inquiry is that one person must rely on another for help with the daily demands of living. The down-to-earth, non-medical, non-expert nature of this help is suggested by these tasks taken from a study of home care for the elderly (Gurland et al., 1978, p. 12):

Assistance or supervision in bathing, grooming, walking, feeding.
Cleaning of incontinence. Toilet training.
Shopping, planning meals, cooking, laundry.
Errands, correspondence, managing cash, advice on personal and financial affairs.
Companionship, sitting services, escort for outside excursions.

Advocacy and intermediation, summoning medical or social help as needed.

Not all dependent people need all these kinds of help. Indeed, the very goals of home care vary considerably and choosing objectives in a particular instance is itself problematic. Is it "cure" or "rehabilitation"? And for which people are these achievable purposes? Is it the prevention of further deterioration and the avoidance of institutionalization? Is it, as with some disabled older people, really a matter of maintaining the person in a familiar, supportive environment under conditions of safety and dignity; that is, good care but with no expectation of "cure"? Or is it the "trend toward caring for the terminally ill at home"?* These are all legitimate and appropriate objectives for different individuals or for the same person at different stages in the course of his or her disability and dependency.

Whatever the purposes may be in a particular family, a great amount of family caring takes place. How much is a matter of very broad estimates at this time, for there is no solid count of the number of physically dependent people living at home nor of the kind or extent of care they receive. Depending on the definitions that are used, various studies have placed the number of such individuals between 2,500,000 and 7,800,000, with several estimates clustering between three and four million. What can be said with assurance is that maintaining the present level of family care and forestalling its erosion or breakdown constitute a large and growing social problem, whether measured by the numbers of people or the financial expenditures involved or by the often unrecognized, hidden social costs.

Family home care is assuming greater prominence and importance in this country primarily because the need for it is increasing rapidly. For example, the elderly, who constitute the largest group at risk, are expected to double in number in the next 50 years, reaching a total of 55 million or 22 percent of the U.S. population. Those 75-85 years of age and those over 85, who will need the

---

*A recent book deals with dying at home with the family and a home care service team providing support to the patient. See Elizabeth R. Pritchard et al., eds. *Home care: Living with Dying,* New York: Columbia University Press, 1979, which gives considerable weight to the problems of middle-age and elderly adults. See also Ida M. Martinson and William F. Henry, "Home Care for Dying Children," *Hastings Center Report,"* April 1980, pp. 5-7.

most care, will increase at a more rapid rate than those below 75 (HCFA, 1981, pp. 10-11). Contributing to the heightened significance of the problem are demographic and ideological changes which Perlman and Giele discuss in the paper that follows and which are likely to reduce the supply of caregivers precisely when the demand will be growing.

This convergence of increased demand and declining supply comes at a critical time in the development of social policy in this country. The tendency of the past 100 years has been for public programs to take on more responsibility for the health and welfare of Americans. The most recent turn, in the past five years, is in the direction of reduced governmental responsibility, a trend that is just beginning to be identified in the papers in this collection.

This recent turn of events can be traced to the worldwide economic recession that came on the heels of the 1973 energy crisis and the zooming price of oil and to rising concern about the level of taxes and the limits of public intervention in social problems. One aspect of this movement in opposition to the almost uninterrupted growth of the Welfare State in this country (and in most Western industrialized nations) has been the pressure to redraw the line between public responsibility and family responsibility, an issue that lies at the very heart of the problem of caring for dependent, disabled people.

The weight of opinion among the writers represented in this collection is on the side of a shared responsibility between the State and the Family, a sharing in which public programs make it possible for families to care for dependent relatives. Even if such a policy were more vigorously implemented than at present, the costs of long-term care are likely to rise substantially. If one assumes a continuation of current policies and trends, "the total burden of long term care, whether provided formally or informally, is certain to increase in the future" (HCFA, 1981, p. 25).

These trends will confront Americans with hard choices. Will they and their political leaders be willing to support larger budgets for home care of the dependent and for assistance to their families? What priority will this receive in the present efforts to cut back social programs and reduce taxes? The question becomes the more politically poignant when one recognizes that few if any of these expenditures can be expected to return people to more self-sufficient roles as earners and taxpayers.

By the very nature of the population at risk—60 percent of

whom are over 65 years of age—home care is primarily concerned
with maintaining an acceptable quality of life for people who are
chronically dependent. The test that some critics of the Welfare
State apply to social programs—will they pay off in financial
returns to the taxpayer—will have mixed results in the case of
home care. Public expenditures for this purpose are primarily in-
vestments in a decent, humane quality of life for millions of Americans, though they may forestall even larger outlays for institutional
care. In any event, these expenditures are not assured of strong
political support in the budget-cutting climate of the 1980s.

Because of the complexities of the problem, it would be useful
to have a framework to help sort out the facts and find their
meaning. The framework should account for critical outcomes and
should illuminate the main issues in family home care. Such a
conceptual scheme is presented in the first paper in the collection
and its main themes are noted here briefly. A useful framework
cannot rest on a single perspective. While the interests of the main
actors—the dependent individuals, their families, and society at
large—can converge under certain circumstances, they can also
compete and conflict with each other under other circumstances.
The organizing scheme must identify these distinct interests.

The framework must also give attention to the dynamics of
home care at two levels—the micro level of the family and its
dependent relative and the macro level at which demographic,
economic, and cultural forces shape the constraints and the opportunities within which family home care operates. Developments
at these two levels are of course closely related: the macro forces
are played out in part through the attitudes and behavior of particular families. Conversely, the aggregate decisions and actions of
family members impart direction and energy to the broad social
changes, as for example the entry into the labor force of more
women, the largest traditional source of home care.

In the light of these considerations, our framework is structured
around five themes or issues:

1. *The adequacy of home care and consequently the quality of
life of the dependent person depend largely on the resources of
the family and the community*. The specific combination of family
caring, formal services, and institutional care that will be best for
the person at risk is problematic. The mix will vary from individual
to individual and from time to time for the same person.

2. *Where the resources of the family are overextended, serious*

*impacts may follow for the dependent person, the family, and ulti-
mately for the community.* This phenomenon of "family burden" is
made painfully clear in this vignette:

> Imagine the plight of a tired mother of six children, all under
> ten years of age, when a physical therapist tells her she must
> exercise her handicapped three-year-old's legs an hour a day.
> It is not surprising that we see evidence of stress in that
> family nor should we be puzzled when she tearfully requests
> removal of the handicapped child from the home. (Skarnulis,
> 1979)

When the burden is too great, the situation is likely to slide toward
one of these outcomes: deterioration of care, institutionalization of
the disabled family member, or breakdown of the family.

3. *The demands inherent in the condition of the dependent
individual and the inputs of the family and of social agencies are
precarious and changeable.* For example, a deterioration in the
physical condition of a disabled person can increase the burden on
his or her family, and this may require the addition of services
from the outside. Or, an increase in the availability of services in a
community may make it possible for certain families to continue to
give care. Likewise, a drop in a family's capacities through unemployment, illness, or divorce can seriously upset an equilibrium
that had earlier been achieved.

These elements are in constant flux. Their changeability has
both positive and negative potentialities. When a family readjusts
to a change in either the condition of the dependent person and/or in
the supportive services—perhaps by rearranging roles and responsibilities within the family—the accommodation can have positive
results all around. But if one element changes and corresponding
adjustments are not forthcoming, the outcome can indeed be negative.

4. *Society's stake lies in protecting the welfare of disabled
individuals and their families and, at the same time, containing the
costs of home care and institutional care.* As society's agents,
health and welfare programs must try to balance these objectives
by coping with the well-known parade of political and organizational problems; typical of these is the effort to make programs
effective in the face of uncertain goals and criteria for success as
well as keeping programs efficient and accountable, yet flexible
and responsive to consumers' needs.

5. *The dynamics of family care at the micro level are significantly influenced by broad developments in American society,
notably by demographic trends, economic and political circumstances, and ideological commitments.* The increase in one-parent
families and the high geographic mobility among American families illustrate the demographic pressures that tend to decrease the
amount of family care available, as do inflation and the cutting
back of social services on which families depend for assistance in
caring for a disabled relative. Our view of the subject must be
broad enough to see the impact of these social changes on the need
for and the provision of home care by American families.

This book is concerned with the issues and themes outlined
above. New data on the prevalence of home care and on the
characteristics of the dependent relatives and their families are
analyzed by Perlman and Giele in Part I. Their analysis relates
variations in family resources to the dependency level of the disabled relative and to a number of socioeconomic characteristics of
the families. A preliminary attempt at assessing the adequacy of
the "fit" for certain types of families is presented, with implications
for policy in this area.

The selections in Part II consider the needs of four types of
dependent persons in relation to the resources of their families.
While the papers take note of the unique problems of each group—
the aged, people with developmental disabilities, mental patients,
and unwed, adolescent mothers—several findings and arguments
of a general nature run through these presentations. The writers
analyze the factors associated with the willingness to provide home
care and attest to the fact that many, many families in fact undertake this task in the face of heavy demands on them.

Two quite different notes are sounded in these papers. Three of
the writers—Horejsi, Segal, and Klerman—take what might be
called an optimistic approach. They feel that if appropriate supportive assistance is provided to families in sufficient quantity,
most families will be able, physically and psychologically, to cope.
Two authors (Farber and Monk) take a more sober, cautious view.

Farber locates the source of the social problem not in the vic-
tims—in this instance, developmentally delayed children, their
parents and siblings—but in the ambivalent signals they receive
from society. They are pushed in one direction toward a life of
"freedom and self-realization" and are pressed in another direction
by the insistence that they assume tremendous responsibilities.

Farber sees in these situations tragedy and pain that he says can never be eliminated, though it may be mitigated by a greater acceptance of the "normality of disappointment." Monk warns us not to expect miracles from family support systems which will not do away with institutional care of the aged people about whom he writes. Moreover, he points out, geographic separation of the generations and declining fertility rates are further depleting the available pool of family resources.

The planning of long-term care entails choices by the individual involved (if he or she is competent to choose), by the family, and by professionals in health and welfare organizations. The choices concern the goals to be sought and the means to be used, that is, whether the site will be the family home, a nursing home, or other institutional setting; the package of services to be delivered, the mix of paid and unpaid help, etc. In the last paper in Part II, Sager asks who makes these choices and what are the consequences when they are made by consumers or by professionals. He found in his investigation that on balance the choices made by all types of participants seemed reasonable. There are direct implications for policy-making in his conclusion that "fears of uncontrollable spending ensuing from patient or family influence over care planning find no support" in his study.

The next group of papers in this collection takes up first the theme of the care-taking role of the American family in the light of broad cultural and economic developments in our history. The very definition of what constitutes dependency (or vulnerability or "otherness"), Demos reminds us, has reflected changing social and economic circumstances since the settlers landed here three centuries ago. The functions of the family have altered (mostly diminished) in ways that affect the care of dependent people. In a reverse mirror image, public provisions (notably the "asylum movement" of the 19th century) have waxed to fit contemporary conditions and ideas.

As for the codification of family responsibility in the law, De Jong makes clear that the caring function *per se*, aside from financial support, has never been explicitly defined by legislators or the courts, though there is a widespread presumption that families should take care of vulnerable relatives especially within the nuclear family. This presumption appears to be less prevalent now than it was earlier in our history.

Family care is now and is likely to continue to be the largest source of care for dependent and disabled people—and should be, judged by humane and economic considerations. In most instances, however, families cannot carry this burden unaided for long periods of time. What are the consequences of public intervention and a division or sharing of the responsibilities between the family and the State? Who should perform what services and who should bear which costs? What forms of financing should be employed? Above all, in terms of broad social policy, does State intervention weaken or strengthen families and does it lead to more or less family caring?

Moroney discusses these questions and concludes that State vs. family responsibility is a misleading dichotomy and that a policy of shared responsibility should guide our collective decisions and actions. The results of policy choices already made are analyzed in the papers on mental retardation and schizophrenia by Morell and Hart respectively. The meager spending on services for retarded children and their families in comparison with expenditures for retarded adults, Morell argues, has favored community-based services for adults at the expense of the deinstitutionalization of children. Similarly, the lack of financial and other supports for the families of schizophrenics living at home has tilted utilization patterns away from home care and toward nursing homes and the revolving doors of mental hospitals.

In the final paper Morris sets forth the constraints and options that should inform policy debate about home-based family care. He places the issues squarely in the context of the questioning of the Welfare State that now pervades public discussion and policy-making in this and other industrial countries. He refers particularly to the ineffectiveness of many public social services and to the abuse of authority by professionals in making vital decisions on a case-by-case basis. To these he adds the practical difficulties of defining today who constitutes a family and who will perform home care tasks, given the shrinkage of available time within the family and the widespread aversion to these chores.

> Most of the tasks with which we will have to deal are un-
> pleasant ones. The vulnerable conditions are not the ones
> which respond to medical or rehabilitative therapy in a rea-
> sonable period of time; they are the problems which persist
> over time and for which the individuals require a great deal
> of physical care and patience. It is just these unpleasant tasks

which families as well as social agencies and medical institutions prefer to off-load to someone else, given an opportunity.

Taking into account these obstacles and difficulties, Morris assesses the merits and the feasibility of five alternative policies for the financing, administration, and delivery of home care.

Our trail through this territory begins, however, in the following paper, with a closer look at the extent of family home care in the United States, at the characteristics of the dependent people and their families, and at some findings on the balance between the needs of the former and the resources of the families.

# An Unstable Triad: Dependents' Demands, Family Resources, Community Supports

Robert Perlman
Janet Z. Giele

On the national level, family home care is a large and growing undertaking. At the household level it is a complex, delicately balanced system that involves trade-offs among the interests of three principal actors—the dependent person, the family, and the community. A model that is useful for understanding these dynamics is presented at the beginning of this chapter. Next, we present new data on the prevalence of family home care in the United States and on the characteristics of the dependent population and their families. Finally, this chapter compares the capacities of caregiving families with the needs of severely, moderately, and mildly dependent family members.

Our model assumes that the key variables in the system are:

1. *the physical and emotional needs and demands* that the dependent person places upon the family;
2. *the material and non-material capacities of the families* to meet the dependent person's needs and simultaneously to fulfill other family functions; and
3. *the availability and use of community resources* such as social services.

A change in any one of these variables, it is assumed, will affect the other elements and will require compensatory adjustments. A conceptual approach similar to this was developed in a study of families in the energy crisis (Perlman and Warren, 1977), where a model was constructed primarily out of crisis theory. In home care, the fulcrum of the system rests on the resources and capacities of the family. A shift either in the demands on the family as a result of a change in the condition of the dependent person or in the use of community resources will necessitate readjustments.

If, for example, an older person living with a family suffers a decline in his or her ability to carry out the usual daily activities, more aid will be needed from the family and/or from other relatives, friends, and neighbors, or from a social agency. Similarly, in the same family, if the care-taking daughter who has remained at home decides to take a full-time job, the caring responsibilities will have to be modified accordingly. If they cannot be rearranged, the outcome may be one or more of the following: a decline in the quality of care and a deterioration in the condition of the parent being cared for; a decrease in the quality of life for the adult child who is torn between two roles; or ultimately a decision to place the older person in an institutional setting.

These assumptions were borne out in the experience of the Family Support Program undertaken by the Community Service Society of New York. The researchers reported (Frankfather et al., 1981, p. 21):

> In slightly fewer than half of the cases, applications were made in response to an abrupt deterioration in the condition of the older person (25 percent), a change in the family (14 percent), or a change in formal home-care services (10 percent). In the last category, the problem typically was the expiration of Medicare financing for services of home health aides.

The family's resources include their financial assets and income, the amount of time they have or are willing to devote to care-taking, the physical and emotional strength of the family members, and their values and attitudes toward this kind of responsibility.

The model calls attention to family adjustments to crises as a process or sequence, beginning with the exploration of possible responses and moving on to a series of tentative adjustments. It is important to understand better than we now do how families initially move into the care-giving role and under what circumstances they withdraw. These dynamics are probably influenced by a family's previous history of crisis management and problem-resolution. Certain families have coped more or less effectively with demands and crises such as the illness or death of a family member or sudden changes in their economic security. They may as a consequence be better prepared to take on and sustain the care of a dependent person than families who have had serious difficulties in dealing with such crises in the past. Still other families have not experienced major crises before they are confronted with the demands of home care and their capabilities are untested. A family's history is only one of the resources it brings to the tasks of caring for a dependent relative. One of the most critical problems in home care is the risk of exhausting these resources as the process extends over time. The result can be "burn-out" for families in which the demands exceed the available resources.

The model outlined above is represented in Figure A.

## MACRO LEVEL FORCES AT WORK

These dynamics at the micro level both reflect and influence broad social forces at the macro level, such as demographic changes and ideological currents. Among the principal developments af-

Figure A

Model of the Family Care System

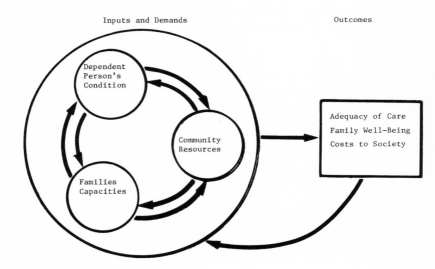

fecting family home care—which are discussed below—are changes in family structure, such as the decreasing size of families and the rise in women's labor force participation. In addition, ethnic, racial, class, and rural-urban differences give some handicapped persons a greater chance of being cared for in the home. Finally, individualistic attitudes and values on the part of some may operate to discourage direct family care, while at the same time there is a growing debate about the extent of responsibility the State should assume for its disabled citizens.

1. *Changing living arrangements.* A remarkable change in living arrangements has been taking place, particularly in the number of older people, especially women, who live alone as primary individuals. Just since 1965, the proportion of females over 65 living in families declined from 63 percent to 56 percent, and the numbers living alone rose by a corresponding amount, from 31 percent to 37 percent (Siegel et al., 1978). In this connection one must note the remarkable sex difference in numbers of old people who live alone. In 1975, 80 percent of older males lived in a family (compared with 56 percent of females), while only 15 percent lived alone as primary individuals. While it might be argued that such changes are the result of a *preference* for privacy and individualism, Kobrin (1976, p. 238) cogently notes that it is primarily the young who prefer such arrangements and that among women over 55, more than half do not.

In relation to family home care, an interesting question to which there is no firm answer is whether persons living alone will have less chance of being cared for by relatives when they are old and disabled. To the extent that living as a primary individual militates against later care by the family, current trends in living arrangements will constitute an additional threat to family home care, especially in the case of older women.

2. *Absent family members.* Comparative studies of institutionalized and non-institutionalized individuals underscore several important differences in the family situations of the two groups. Among the elderly, especially, many more of the institutionalized persons lack family members to care for them. They are more likely to be single, widowed, or childless. In addition a disproportionate number of those in institutions who need personal care only (as opposed to skilled nursing) are evidently there because they have no family with whom to live (NCHS, 1969, 1973; S.J. Brody et al., 1978; Giele, 1981, p. 6-7).

Such findings raise a question: will the forces that contribute to the lack of relatives, including siblings, be on the rise or on the wane in coming generations? Smaller family size and childlessness seem likely to decrease family resources to provide home care.

Similar questions can be raised about the effects of present high divorce rates or widowhood. Any estimate at this point must be highly speculative. Nevertheless, on the basis of what is presently known, it can be said that the person without a spouse or child or sibling to fall back on is much more vulnerable to institutionalization.

3. *Women's labor force participation.* Rising employment of women threatens the capacity for family home care another way: it diminishes the pool of available caretakers, traditionally middle-aged women, who have tended the disabled and handicapped. Townsend (1957) and Rosenmayr (1977) have documented the preference of older people for care by daughters; Blenkner (1963) and E.M. Brody (1978) have similarly suggested that in the United States it is primarily middle-aged women who carry the chief responsibility for family home care. Yet Moroney (1976) has shown that the middle-aged female caretaker pool is shrinking. Women have compressed their child-bearing into the years before they are thirty and changed their expectations from lifelong housewifery to employment outside the home (Giele, 1978, p. 147). Few countervailing forces are evident that can shift this trend in the opposite direction.

4. *Race, class, and income differences.* In minority groups some of the trends noted above, such as absence of next-of-kin, are compounded with poorer health status, poverty, and inadequate housing to produce severe needs for home care but more difficulties in providing it. Across all income groups, for example, nonwhite elderly had more than twice as many bed disability days as whites in 1974 (Congressional Budget Office, 1977, p. 4). Moreover, nonwhites have lower median incomes and therefore fewer material resources for providing family care.

Nonwhite persons are also less likely to have family members who are available to care for them. The *1976 Survey of Institutionalized Persons* reports that almost twice as many blacks (18 percent) report no living next-of-kin as whites (10 percent) (U.S. Bureau of Census, 1978a, p. 237).

Finally, a much smaller proportion of the nonwhite population lives in suburban areas (roughly one-third the proportion of whites). Nearly three-fifths of blacks live in central city areas (U.S. Senate

1971, p. viii). To the extent that suburban dependents are more likely to receive help from family as Mahoney (1977) has shown, and urban handicapped people are less likely to do so, the nonwhite minority population faces even more severe threats to family home care than the white majority. What has not been carefully studied, though it may be an important element, is the variation in norms and expectations concerning family care among groups differentiated by race, ethnicity, religion, and social class.

5. *Rural, suburban, and urban variations.* The growing urbanism of American society, while it provides more services in urban places, also has the paradoxical effect of decreasing the opportunities for family home care. Rosenmayr (1977), in an extensive survey of the elderly in Austria, found marked rural-urban contrasts. In small communities (up to 2,000 population) only 14 percent of the elderly expected to be cared for by non-family members or by no one. In Vienna, however, 20 percent of the males (75-99) and 37 percent of the females (75-99) expected to be cared for by people outside the family or by no one.

In the United States Mahoney (1977) reanalyzed Harris poll data from 1974 that asked elderly people how much help they needed and how much they received from relatives. He found that rural and suburban elderly were more likely to get help from non-family members than those living in urban locations.

6. *Individualistic values.* Besides demographic trends that suggest structural threats to family home care, there are shifts in attitudes and values that portend a more individualistic society where the family's sense of responsibility for care of its members may be attenuated. Barbara Silverstone (1978) has said that more middle-aged people today believe that they should have the opportunity to enjoy "a life of their own." Alvin Schorr (1980) has documented the change that took place since 1950 in national policy toward the aged. When programs such as Social Security and Medicare adopted their present eligibility requirements, they accepted a shift from personal filial responsibility on the part of an older person's children to universalized societal responsibility for the older generation.

In an advanced urban society, a high degree of individuation may be altogether appropriate. Treas (1975) has noted that good parents frequently have a "developmental stake" in their children's establishment of separate living arrangements and geographical mobility even if this sometimes puts great distances between family members. Nevertheless, such patterns of behavior that are adaptive earlier in the life cycle may diminish the likelihood of joint living arrangements at a later time when parents need care. As pointed out above, it is also not clear how these individualistic values are distributed among groups differentiated by income, race and ethnicity, and religion.

7. *Countervailing forces on behalf of family care.* In sum, the natural or traditional willingness and ability of families to care for their disabled members may in the future be dramatically altered. The present volume of family care is impressive, however, and several positive forces should be noted that potentially may help to sustain it.

The contributions of disabled people to the family could gain in importance. Townsend (1957) portrayed the many services old people performed for their families—making meals, looking after children, sometimes contributing financially. An emphasis on the reciprocal nature of the care-taking arrangement could fundamentally reinforce the traditional willingness of the family to give care.

Changes in labor force participation that have taken women out of the home could also operate to support family care, if other potential caretakers can be tapped, e.g., youth or men who retire early. In addition, employment of such persons in homemaker services could help to sustain care where institutionalization might be the only other reasonable alternative.

Finally, changes in living and housing arrangements to permit "intimacy at a distance" might in the long run sustain family care by subsidizing additions to homes or other similar facilities that encourage the disabled individual's independence as well as family responsibility.

Whether the forces working on behalf of family care or the countervailing pressures will in the long run have more effect can only be seen by close examination of trends in living arrangements of dependent and disabled people. The following section examines estimates of the current prevalence of family home care in the United States and describes some of the characteristics of the dependent population and their families.

## PREVALENCE OF FAMILY HOME CARE

It would be useful for policy-making and program planning to know the prevalence of family home care in the United States and to have information on the characteristics of the dependent individuals and their families, but very little is known with any certainty. The estimates that are available are based on the individuals who depend on home care from their families. But before one can describe these people, it is essential to understand what phenomena the figures are counting. We must begin, therefore, with words and concepts before we look at numbers.

Impairment, disability, handicap, limitation, dependency—the words denote quite different situations and vary according to the purpose at hand and the organizational and professional context.[1] For example, disability is described as "primarily a medical problem, a health-related inability to work" by researchers concerned essentially with the employment and income of adults of working age (Berkowitz et al., 1976, p. 7). What is important for us to recognize is that the definitions refer, more often implicitly than explicitly, to one or more of the following aspects of a person's physical limitation: (1) its cause, (2) whether and how it can be alleviated or remedied, (3) the person's presumed ability to perform specific functions, or (4) its impact on the person's actual activities.

Here we are more interested in the effects of a disabling condition on the actual functioning of individuals and in the impact on their families than we are in the etiology, or the remediability of the condition. Most surveys do not define the problem in this way and, with a few exceptions, we must rely on estimates that do not indicate the need for personal care, do not specify whether the person lives at home, or if so, whether alone or with his or her family.

Subject to these caveats, two estimates are cited here and others are in a note at the end of the chapter.[2] Writing only about *the elderly,* Morris and Youket state that "over 3 million family units . . . provide major physical, personal or financial help to their disabled elderly living outside of institutions." They also refer to an HEW estimate that *some* of the 3.6 to 7.8 million *disabled adults* in 1978 received informal care through family or friends (Morris and Youket, 1980, pp. 1-4). Other estimates of the number of families who provide home care cluster between 3 and 5 million. In short, only fragments and approximations are available on the volume of family care and the characteristics of the people who give and receive it.

Fortunately, in its 1976 *Survey of Income and Education* (SIE) the Census Bureau included several questions about disability and specifically about the need for personal care in 181,000 American families, although this was incidental to other purposes. What the SIE lacks by way of detail on dependency and family care is, in our view, more than compensated by the fact that there seems to be no other source with so much useful data on so many individuals and families, even though the findings are subject to the limitations of self-reported data. Boggs and Henney (n.d.) comment that the SIE "is the most reliable source now available for estimating the developmentally disabled population in the United States" based on functional limitations.

We have selected from the SIE data a population who *usually or frequently "need help from others in looking after personal needs, such as eating, dressing, undressing, or personal hygiene"* or who frequently *"need help from others to go outdoors or to get around outside their home."* * We refer to this population as *severely dependent.* Using this definition, some 2,342,000 *severely dependent* persons can be identified in the survey. Some 18 percent of these individuals live alone, a considerably higher proportion than 7.1 percent of the general population who live alone. This leaves 1.9 million severely dependent persons living with one or more members of their families and, presumably, receiving care at home.

There is considerable overlap among those people who frequently need help with personal care and those who frequently need help getting about outside their homes. In the SIE severely dependent group, 60 percent said they needed *both* kinds of assistance; 33 percent said they needed help only with mobility and 7 percent said they required only personal aid.

It must be emphasized that these 1.9 million individuals are the *most dependent* people living with their families and that, in lesser degrees, many others are probably the beneficiaries of family home care. For example, the SIE survey identified an additional 1.2 million persons who could not attend school or work or could work only occasionally. The 1.9 million severely dependent plus the 1.2 million unable to go to school or work regularly are part of a much larger population of 28 million people who are limited in their daily activities, though not necessarily in need of physical assistance.

These 28 million *persons with activity limitations* consist of individuals who have a physical, emotional, or mental condition that limits their ability to engage in activities appropriate for their ages, such as attending school, playing, going to work, or working

---

*This corresponds to the definition of a severely dependent person used by DeJong and Sager, i.e. someone who scores less than 61 out of 100 on the Barthel Index "based on the amount of help a person needs with self-care and mobility." (DeJong and Sager, 1977)

around the house. Within this population there are certainly many who must call upon their families for varying degrees of assistance. However, we shall concentrate our analysis of the prevalence of family home care in the population who frequently need personal help, that is, the severely dependent, who make more substantial demands on their families than the others.

The severely dependent represent 1.1 percent of the total United States population, according to the SIE data, and their families constitute 3.4 percent of all families, not taking into account the small proportion of families with more than one dependent person. While these percentages do not accurately measure the prevalence of family home care, they do identify a population that is at the core of the issues discussed here. In describing them, wherever possible we shall compare them with the general population of the United States and, at points, with the 28 million with activity limitations.

The outstanding characteristic of the severely dependent is the predominance of older people. The disability prevalence rate of persons 65 and older as shown in Table 1 is ten times that of people in the 18-64 year old group and 25 times more than that of children and teenagers.

Females are overrepresented among the dependent receiving family care, accounting for 57.8 percent of the total. This is especially evident among women over 65 years of age, who constitute one-third of all severely dependent people, compared with older men who make up only one-sixth of the total. This close association of age, disability, and dependency was to be expected. Schorr, for example, has estimated that three to four million of the elderly are disabled and are not capable of independent daily living and that about two-thirds of them are in their own homes (Schorr, 1980). It is also well known that a disproportionate number of the elderly are women.

The SIE data throw additional light on the physically dependent elderly. They indicate that while one-fourth of the dependent elderly live alone, half live in a two-person household and another fourth live in households of three or more people. It is worth noting that 5.6 percent of the elderly who live alone are severely dependent, in contrast to 6.6 percent of those living with relatives who are severely dependent. In other words, three-quarters of the elderly who are severely dependent live with members of their families who are available, in different degrees, to assist them. This care is

TABLE 1

Severely Dependent Noninstitutionalized Persons in U.S., 1975 by Age and Race

| | Severely Dependent (thousands) | Number per 1,000 persons in each age or ethnic group |
|---|---|---|
| **Age** | | |
| 3-17 | 153 | 2.6 |
| 18-64 | 771 | 5.8 |
| 65+ | 1,419 | 63.3 |
| | | |
| **Race & Ethnicity** | | |
| White and other | 1,984 | 10.9 |
| Black | 288 | 12.1 |
| Hispanic | 71 | 6.3 |
| | | |
| ALL AGES | 2,343[1] | 10.8 |

[1]This includes 423,452 persons living alone or 18.1 percent of the total, compared with 7.1 percent for the general population. No single-person households were identified for people under 25 years of age. Some 10.5 percent of those 25-64 lived alone and 24.7 percent of those 65 and over lived alone.

Source:  Authors' tabulation of data from U.S. Department of Commerce, Bureau of the Census, Survey of Income and Education, 1976; Current Population Reports, Series P-25, No. 614, 1975, and Series P-20, No. 292, 1976, and Statistical Abstract of the United States, 1976, Table 28.

often provided for extended periods of time. Among those cared for at home, according to one study, 25 percent received care for more than five years. Nearly three-fourths of those 75 years of age and older received home care for more than a year (Maddox, 1975).

People in the 18-64 year age group have a much lower rate of dependency than the elderly. These people, who constitute slightly more than half the U.S. population, have only half the number of severely dependents as the elderly.

The numbers and the proportion of pre-school and school age children (ages 3 to 17) who were identified as severely dependent in the SIE are relatively small, but they may be increasing. They amount to only 3 out of every 1000 American children and teen-agers. But there are indications that the most disabled children are being cared for in larger numbers by their families. Morell (below) reports that two-thirds of the families with substantially retarded children in the United States are now caring for the child at home, i.e., 160,000 children. More and more infants are brought home from hospitals with serious chronic illnesses or handicapping conditions. The Children's Hospital Medical Center in Boston has initiated a "home intervention project" to assist parents in coping with incapacitated children (Brownstein and Berkley, 1979).

Turning from age and sex to race, prevalence rates for whites and blacks are generally similar, though a bit higher among blacks over 18 years of age. However, the overall rate for Hispanics is roughly half that of the other two groups, a finding that at first seems implausible, since, within the major age groups, Hispanics' rates are very close to those of the general population. The explanation lies primarily in the fact that the age structure of the Hispanic population differs markedly from Americans as a whole; they have proportionately many more young people (whose rates for dependency are low) and a much smaller elderly group (whose rates are high).

Being dependent and living with one's family is a situation that varies considerably in terms of specific disabilities and diseases. Before describing severely dependent Americans in these terms, it is important to note the extent of multiple disabilities. One-fourth of the people with an activity limitation—28 million in the SIE—reported having more than one disabling condition. Some 16 percent had two conditions reported and 10 percent were said to have three or more conditions that limited their activities. What are the prevalence rates of severe dependency among the activity-limited population and how do these vary by age? Table 2 shows that mental retardation and speech impairment are significant among persons under 25 and that orthopedic handicaps peak in the 18-24 year old group. Dependency increases with age for people who report hearing impairments, blindness, spine or back troubles, and particularly cardiac conditions. Generally, rates for males and females are quite similar. It must be noted again that these diagnoses were given by household respondents in a Census Bureau survey and are subject to reporting errors.

The SIE provides information on the work and school status of the most dependent people. Respondents were asked what they had been doing most of the week previous to the survey. The responses, shown in Table 3, indicate that approximately half of the school-

TABLE 2

Severely Dependent Persons by Age and Type of Condition* (in percent)

| | Male | | | | | Female | | | | |
|---|---|---|---|---|---|---|---|---|---|---|
| | 3-13 | 14-17 | 18-24 | 25-64 | 65+ | 3-13 | 14-17 | 18-24 | 25-64 | 65+ |
| Mentally retarded | 54 | 66 | 51 | 25 | 3 | 48 | 63 | 67 | 20 | 1 |
| Hard of hearing | 6 | 3 | 2 | 10 | 22 | 8 | 8 | 3 | 3 | 21 |
| Deaf | 6 | - | - | - | 3 | 0 | 8 | 4 | 2 | 6 |
| Speech impairment | 35 | 6 | 21 | 13 | 11 | 15 | 29 | 18 | 10 | 4 |
| Blindness or difficulty seeing | 8 | - | 8 | 17 | 27 | 13 | 5 | 16 | 20 | 28 |
| Serious emotional disturbance | 6 | 6 | 14 | 10 | 6 | 12 | 2 | 15 | 9 | 3 |
| Crippled (orthopedic handicap) | 27 | 44 | 38 | 30 | 21 | 26 | 29 | 30 | 29 | 25 |
| Arthritis or rheumatism | 2 | - | 2 | 19 | 31 | 0 | 4 | 0 | 31 | 51 |
| Trouble with back or spine | 5 | 5 | 12 | 24 | 15 | 13 | 12 | 2 | 21 | 17 |
| Heart trouble | 5 | 3 | 2 | 25 | 47 | 9 | 9 | 0 | 18 | 40 |
| Chronic nervous disorder | 3 | 2 | 4 | 15 | 8 | 15 | 7 | 2 | 14 | 8 |
| Respiratory disorder | 9 | - | 8 | 15 | 28 | 20 | 12 | 2 | 9 | 9 |
| Digestive disorder | - | - | 4 | 9 | 9 | 0 | 0 | 0 | 9 | 12 |

AGE

*The columns do not add to 100 percent since there are individuals with multiple handicaps.

Source: Authors' tabulation of unpublished data from U.S. Department of Commerce, Bureau of the Census, Survey of Income and Education, 1976.

TABLE 3

Work and School Status of Severely Dependent by Age and Sex, 1975

| | Male | | | | Female | | | |
|---|---|---|---|---|---|---|---|---|
| | 14-17 | 18-24 | 25-64 | 65+ | 14-17 | 18-24 | 25-64 | 65+ |
| Unable to work | 16 | 46 | 64 | 37 | 18 | 43 | 48 | 42 |
| At school | 51 | 25 | 1 | - | 57 | 21 | 2 | - |
| Working | 1 | 7 | 8 | 1 | 2 | 9 | 4 | - |
| Keeping house | - | - | - | 1 | - | 9 | 30 | 25 |
| Other* | 32 | 22 | 27 | 61 | 23 | 18 | 16 | 33 |
| Total | 100 | 100 | 100 | 100 | 100 | 100 | 100 | 100 |

*Includes retired, with job but not at work, and looking for work.

Source: Authors' tabulation of unpublished data, U.S. Department of Commerce, Bureau of the Census, Survey of Income and Education, 1976.

age children were not in school and that almost half to two-thirds of the people 18 to 64 were unable to work. Only a small percentage of people in the post-school years were at work. Among those who were asked why they were not looking for work, half of the 18-24 year old respondents said it was because of poor health; more than 90 percent of those over 64 gave the same reason.

Some of the implications for the dependent individuals and their families are plain. The presence of school-age children at home necessitated, for many families, someone in the home to care for them. A similar assumption seems reasonable for many of the elderly. The working-age group presents an additional problem: not only were they at home, in some instances requiring personal aid, but many were not earning and were thus not contributing to the family's income. It is this combined effect of disability and dependency that has a serious impact on the family. Families with a disabled adult of working age "lose" their earnings at the very time that many of them face increased expenses.

We ought now to look more closely at the resources that families bring to the care of a dependent person, specifically at their economic situation and the number of people in the family. The latter is a crude measure of the time and energy that may be available for home care.

Families caring for a dependent relative are smaller than the population at large, as Table 4 makes clear. Dependent people live in two-person families to a greater extent than the general population and they live in families of four or more to a lesser extent. Part of this effect is due to the large numbers of elderly among the disabled who are likely to live in smaller families in part because of their age. To the degree that fewer family members means less time and energy available for providing personal care, care-providing families are again at a disadvantage: they have fewer resources than the population at large but their circumstances demand more than is demanded of the typical family. In terms of race and ethnicity, the data indicate that black and Hispanic families are larger than white families, but this advantage in numbers may be offset by their lower economic resources.

The lower economic status of care-giving families compared with all families in the United States is apparent from Table 5. Half the care-giving families fall below $10,000 in income, in contrast to approximately one-third in the general population. By the same token, only 30 percent of families with dependent people living at home have incomes in excess of $15,000, in comparison with 40 percent of all families.

TABLE 4

Size of Family of Dependent Persons (SIE) and for U.S. Population, 1975

| | SIE Dependent* | U.S. Population White | Black | Hispanic |
|---|---|---|---|---|
| Two persons | 48 | 38.5 | 29.4 | 23.2 |
| Three persons | 22 | 21.6 | 22.7 | 22.5 |
| Four persons | 13 | 19.9 | 17.8 | 20.5 |
| Five persons or more | 17 | 20.0 | 30.1 | 33.8 |
| Percent | 100 | 100.0 | 100.0 | 100.0 |

Note: The 18 percent of all severely dependent people who live alone are not included in the table. This compares with 7 percent for the general population.

*Based on a 10 percent sample of the disabled in the SIE.

Source: Authors' tabulation of unpublished data, U.S. Department of Commerce, Bureau of the Census, *Survey of Income and Education, 1976*; *Current Population Reports*, Series P-20, No. 292, 1976.

TABLE 5

Family Income of Dependent Persons (SIE)
and of Total U.S. Population, 1974-75

| Family Income | All U.S. Families 1974 | Families With Dependent Members, SIE |
|---|---|---|
| Under $5,000 | 13.1 | 25.9 |
| $5,000-9,999 | 22.7 | 25.7 |
| $10,000-14,999 | 24.3 | 19.0 |
| $15,000 or more | 39.8 | 29.4 |
| | 99.9 | 100.0 |

Sources: U.S. Department of Commerce, Bureau of the Census, Current Population Reports, Series P-60, No. 101, 1976, and authors' tabulation of a 10 percent sample of dependent persons, unpublished data, U.S. Department of Commerce, Bureau of the Census, Survey of Income and Education, 1976.

Proportionately more severely dependent persons live in poverty than is the case with the United States population as a whole, except among the elderly. For dependent persons under 65 years of age, the percentage in poverty varies between 17 and 24, while for the population at large the corresponding percentages range from 7 to 16, depending on the age group. On the other hand, among the severely dependent over 65, only 8 percent live below the poverty level, compared with 14 percent for the elderly population as a whole. The relatively higher economic status among the dependent elderly may reflect a greater measure of public support that comes to them as a result of their dependence and disabilities.

## SIE FAMILIES WHO PROVIDE CARE

Families who care for the handicapped may be smaller and poorer than other families, but it is possible that such a generalization, without going deeper, would distort the picture. It may be, for example, that families of the handicapped have made adjustments in their family time and used their resources in such a fashion as to enable them to give care. One might imagine that these families are in certain respects "stronger" than the average, with advantages in structure, size, or time resources that permit them to adapt to their extra burdens. If they do not have such resources, the handicapped member may no longer live with them. Put another way, an ecological theory would suggest that families find a balance between demands and resources. Some are able to provide needed help entirely by themselves. Others need supplemental supports from outside sources. Still others in some instances are forced to give up care of the disabled member.

There are three major tests of such a theory, and all are indirect. First, one can compare characteristics of the families who give care with those families in the U.S. population who do not have a disabled member. Second, one can compare the home-care families with those families whose members live in institutions. Finally, it is possible to compare families within the "home care" group by examining differences which may exist between the families of the mildly, moderately, or severely disabled. The analysis described here is based only on the first and third types of comparison.[3]

Table 6 shows the screening questions we used to identify the dependent population in the 1976 *Survey of Income and Education* (SIE) and to make distinctions among three levels of disability. While most of the questions called for yes or no answers, the items on school attendance, personal care, and mobility gave an opportunity to tap gradations of severity. As shown in Table 6, a combination of such answers was used to designate mild, moderate, and severe levels of dependency.[4] Moreover, the selection of a representative sample of mildly to severely dependent persons enables more detailed descriptions not only of the handicapped but also of their families. We were able to examine type and size of family, total family income, the amount of family time available for caregiving, and various sources of income. What emerges from these findings is a complex but in some ways encouraging picture that reveals family strengths and resources for giving care as well as the need for more outside help in some instances.

### Family Capacities: Size, Structure, and Available Time

As already shown in earlier sections of this paper, families of the handicapped do display certain deficits compared with the general population. On the average they tend to be smaller; they tend to have lower incomes. It is also true, however, according to our conceptual model that families cannot care for their handi-

TABLE 6

Questions in the SIE Used in Selecting Handicapped or
Dependent Population and in Defining Three
Levels of Dependency

| Item No. | Question | Ages Applicable | Assigned level of disability | | |
|---|---|---|---|---|---|
| | | | Mild | Moderate | Severe |
| 60 | Condition limits regular school work | 14-17 | yes | | |
| 60A | Usually able to attend school | 14-17 | | cannot attend | |
| 61 | Condition limits sports, games | 14-17 | yes | | |
| 63A | Condition limits school work | 18-25 | yes | | |
| 64 | Condition limits kind or amount of work | 18-64 | yes | | |
| 66 | Condition prevents working | 18-64 | | yes | |
| 66A | Able to work only occasionally or irregularly because of health | 18-64 | | yes | |
| 67 | Condition limits work around house | 65+ | yes | | |
| 68 | Needs help in eating, dressing, etc. | 14+ | rarely | | frequently |
| 69 | Needs help to go outdoors | 14+ | rarely | | frequently |
| 89 | Condition limits ability to play games | 5-13 | yes | | |
| Number of Dependent persons (a 10% sample of all 52,380 SIE "handicapped") | | N=5,238 | 3396 | 1445 | 397 |
| Dependent persons as percent of total population of 440,000 individuals in the SIE. | | 11.9% | 8% | 3% | 1% |

capped members unless they have certain capacities or resources
on which they can draw. One would expect that such families
somehow actively adjust to provide needed care. Or perhaps families are able to continue home care of the disabled only if their
initial structure or natural adaptation is adequate to the tasks demanded of them. In any case we would expect that, whatever the
process, the outcomes observed would be in some sense descriptive
only of the "survivors," that is, the families who at the moment

of the survey provided the family environment in which disabled persons could live.

One question to ask then, is what characteristics, if any, distinguish the families in which disabled persons live. Are these families somehow different in size and composition? Table 7 shows median family size by severity of handicap when age of the handicapped person and household structure are held constant. What seems most notable about this table is that within each age group family size is fairly similar across handicap levels. Husband-wife families have a median size of about 5 where the handicapped member is less than 19 years old, and about 4 where the disabled member is 19 to 40 years of age. The size is slightly smaller in

TABLE 7

Median Family Size by Age and Disability Level and
Family Type of Handicapped Person, SIE 1976

| Age of Handicapped Person | | Disability Level | |
|---|---|---|---|
| | | Mild | Moderate & Severe |
| Under 19 | M-FHH | 5.1 | 4.9 |
| | FHH | 3.7 | 2.6 |
| | MHH | 5.1 | -- |
| 19-40 | M-FHH | 4.1 | 3.9 |
| | FHH | 2.5 | 2.8 |
| | MHH | 1.2 | 1.3 |
| 41-54 | M-FHH | 3.4 | 3.2 |
| | FHH | 2.1 | 2.2 |
| | MHH | 1.2 | 1.2 |
| 55-64 | M-FHH | 2.3 | 2.2 |
| | FHH | 1.3 | 1.3 |
| | MHH | 1.3 | 1.2 |
| 65-74 | M-FHH | 2.1 | 2.2 |
| | FHH | 1.1 | 1.3 |
| | MHH | 1.2 | -- |
| 75+ | M-FHH | 2.2 | 2.7 |
| | FHH | 1.2 | 1.5 |
| | MHH | 1.2 | 1.7 |

M-FHH is a household with male and female heads.
FHH is a female-only headed household.
MHH is a male-only headed household.

Source:  Authors' tabulation of unpublished data from the Survey of Income and Education, 1976. Based on 5,238 unweighted cases, a 10 percent sample of the disabled in the SIE.

TABLE 8

Family Type by Age and Disability Level of Handicapped Person, SIE 1976

| Age of Handicapped Person | | Disability Level | | | | | |
|---|---|---|---|---|---|---|---|
| | | Mild | | Moderate | | Severe | |
| | | Number | Percent | Number | Percent | Number | Percent |
| Under 19 | M-FHH | 569 | 81 | 11 | 79 | 16 | 76 |
| | FHH | 122 | 17 | 2 | 14 | 5 | 24 |
| | MHH | 9 | 2 | 1 | 7 | 0 | 0 |
| 19-40 | M-FHH | 410 | 75 | 203 | 70 | 23 | 72 |
| | FHH | 96 | 17 | 75 | 26 | 8 | 25 |
| | MHH | 43 | 8 | 10 | 3 | 1 | 3 |
| 41-54 | M-FHH | 377 | 79 | 318 | 70 | 34 | 74 |
| | FHH | 65 | 14 | 106 | 23 | 11 | 24 |
| | MHH | 32 | 7 | 33 | 7 | 1 | 2 |
| 55-64 | M-FHH | 292 | 81 | 493 | 72 | 37 | 76 |
| | FHH | 52 | 14 | 140 | 20 | 7 | 14 |
| | MHH | 18 | 5 | 53 | 8 | 5 | 10 |
| 65-74 | M-FHH | 502 | 65 | 0 | | 62 | 66 |
| | FHH | 211 | 27 | 0 | | 31 | 33 |
| | MHH | 63 | 8 | 0 | | 1 | 1 |
| 75+ | M-FHH | 270 | 50 | 0 | | 79 | 51 |
| | FHH | 210 | 39 | 0 | | 59 | 38 |
| | MHH | 55 | 10 | 0 | | 17 | 11 |
| | Total | 3396 | | 1445 | | 397 | |
| All ages | M-FHH | | 71% | | 71% | | 63% |
| | FHH | | 22% | | 22% | | 30% |
| | MHH | | 6% | | 7% | | 6% |

U.S. percentages 1975,          M-FHH     65%
Masnick & Bane, p. 57          FHH       24%
                              MHH       11%

Note:  M-FHH  =  Male and female headed Household
       FHH    =  Female only headed Household
       MHH    =  Male only headed Household

Source:  Authors' tabulation of unpublished data from the Survey of Income and
         Education, 1976. Based on 5,238 unweighted cases, a 10 percent sample
         of the disabled in the SIE.

each succeeding age group but never varies more than a few tenths
of a percentage point between handicap levels in the same age
group.

Table 8 shows household structure when families of dependent
persons of the same age and level of dependency are compared.
The three major household types are: (1) those headed by a husband
and wife (M-FHH); (2) those headed by a female (FHH); and (3)
those headed by a male (MHH). What is most striking is that except
for families where the dependent person is over 65, *more husband-*

*wife families (72 to 76 percent) are found among the care-giving families than in the population at large (65 percent).*

Among all households in the United States in 1975, various estimates have put the ratio of husband-wife families at 65 to 62 percent (if primary individuals and single-person households are included) (Masnick and Bane, 1980, pp. 57, 87, 186-187; Barrett, 1979, p. 12). To the extent that single headship or living alone as a primary individual is a sign of limited family resources or greater vulnerability, the higher rate of two-parent families or husband-wife headship can perhaps be taken as a sign of relatively greater family strength and capacity among families of the handicapped. Just what the process is that results in these differentials is not known to us. One possibility is that proportionately more of the single-headed families eventually must give up the care of the handicapped person. Another and perhaps related possibility is that in the case of divorce, widowhood, or separation, kin groups may send the handicapped member to aunts, uncles, grandparents, or siblings who have the family resources that enable them to provide care.

Also of interest in the findings on family structure are similarities and differences between handicap levels. There is virtually no difference in percent of mildly and moderately disabled who live in husband-wife, female, or male-headed families. Among the severely handicapped the proportion of female-headed families does rise because of an interaction with age. The single largest group of severely handicapped are over 75, and in this group only half of all families are headed by both a male and a female. Among the severely handicapped under age 65, however, fully 74 percent are found in households headed by couples, again a figure considerably higher than the overall national average for households in the pre-retirement age groups.

These small clues to the strengths of care-giving families emerge into full-blown evidence from an analysis of family time assets. We devised a rough gauge of aggregate demands on family time—designated by "negative" values—and the family's combined time resources with which to meet the demands, designated by "positive" values. A dependent person was assigned a value of $-1$ if he or she were mildly dependent, $-2$ if moderately dependent, and $-4$ if severely dependent. The time score of each of the other individuals in the family was assigned as follows and then summed:

| | |
|---|---|
| Person under age 6 | $-2$ |
| Person age 6-13 | $-1$ |
| Person engaged in housekeeping | $+2$ |
| Person over 13 working less than 21 hours per week and not regularly in school | $+2$ |
| Other | $+1$ |

For example, in a family consisting of (1) a severely dependent person, (2) a working mother, and (3) a 14-year-old in school, the first person would have a score of $-4$, the second a score of $+1$ and the third a score of $+1$. The overall family time score would be $-2$, indicating a deficit in "time assets."

A calculation of family time potential was thus derived by summing the "individual time" of each of the non-handicapped members and subtracting from that figure a certain number of points depending on severity of the handicapped member's disability. The figures resulted in a range from minus ten ($-10$) to plus ten ($+10$).

Using this family time measure, we see in Table 9 that "positive" family time assets are surprisingly similar across handicap levels when age and family structure are held constant. In addition it is evident in the husband-wife families across all handicapped groups and in the male-headed families of the mildly handicapped that family time assets clearly increase with age of the handicapped person. But in the female-headed households age does not have the same positive effect.

Table 9 also makes quite evident that female-headed households have much smaller time assets at their disposal than the husband-wife families. Where the clear majority of husband-wife households have positive time available in almost every age group and handicap level, exactly the opposite is true for the households headed by a male or female only. Among the mildly handicapped, regardless of age group, for example, 70 percent of all households headed by both husband and wife have positive time available. This figure compares with only 21 percent of the female-headed households and 20 percent of the male-headed households.

The difference in family time assets by handicap level becomes even more dramatic when particular family types are examined more closely. Table 10 presents time resources with size and family type controlled. In both husband-wife families and female-headed families there is a striking *positive* association between amount of

TABLE 9

Percent of Families with Positive Time Assets
by Age, Disability Level, and Family Type of
Handicapped Person, SIE 1976

| Age of Handicapped Person | | Disability Level | | |
|---|---|---|---|---|
| | | M i l d | M o d e r a t e | S e v e r e |
| 18 and under | M-FHH | 62.1 | 54.6 | 56.4 |
| | FHH | 38.5 | 50.0 | 60.0 |
| | MHH | 11.1 | -- | -- |
| 19-40 | M-FHH | 47.2 | 42.4 | 56.3 |
| | FHH | 29.2 | 37.2 | 75.0 |
| | MHH | 16.3 | 16.3 | -- |
| 41-54 | M-FHH | 73.6 | 70.2 | 73.5 |
| | FHH | 47.7 | 39.5 | 36.4 |
| | MHH | 21.9 | 24.3 | -- |
| 55-64 | M-FHH | 78.2 | 69.1 | 72.9 |
| | FHH | 28.8 | 23.6 | 42.9 |
| | MHH | 16.8 | 15.1 | 40.0 |
| 65-74 | M-FHH | 83.9 | -- | 85.6 |
| | FHH | 15.2 | -- | 23.8 |
| | MHH | 25.4 | -- | -- |
| 75 and over | M-FHH | 88.4 | -- | 81.1 |
| | FHH | 16.8 | -- | 40.6 |
| | MHH | 20.0 | -- | 52.9 |

Note:  M-FHH = Male and Female headed Household
       FHH   = Female only headed Household
       MHH   = Male only headed Household

Source:  Authors' tabulation of unpublished data from the Survey of Income and
         Education, 1976. Based on 5,238 unweighted cases, a 10 percent sample
         of the disabled in the SIE.

time available and severity of disability. More of the families with mildly handicapped members show negative time potential, and more of the families with severely handicapped members show positive time potential.

At first such a finding may seem counter-intuitive because one automatically thinks of the more burdened families as worse off. But on further reflection the correlation between time potential and disability level appears to confirm one element of our conceptual model as shown in Figure B. Where the dependent person's needs are greater, there is a tendency for the family to have greater potential (at least in available time) for meeting those needs.

How does such a correlation come about? Perhaps the key factor is age of family members. Positive time available is positively correlated with age of the handicapped member and negatively correlated with presence of young children. Severity of disability is also positively correlated with age. It may be that families decide not to have any more children if they have a disabled member, or within the kinship group, care of the disabled person may be shifted to a household unit where there are no young children present. Still another factor likely to be correlated with age is the presence of retired persons, those working part-time, and women whose employment status is housekeeper. Thus the elderly who

TABLE 10

Family Time Potential by Family Type and Disability
Level of Handicapped Member, in Percentages of
Families with Time Deficits and Assets,
SIE, 1976

Husband-Wife Families (3 or more members)

| Family Time Potential | Disability Level of Handicapped Member | | |
|---|---|---|---|
| | Mild | Moderate | Severe |
| Deficit (-10 to -1) | 26.4 | 27.5 | 15.8 |
| Zero | 13.2 | 12.5 | 9.5 |
| Asset (+1 to +10) | 60.0 | 59.9 | 74.7 |

Female-Headed Families (2 or more members)

| Family Time Potential | Disability Level of Handicapped Member | | |
|---|---|---|---|
| | Mild | Moderate | Severe |
| Deficit (-10 to -1) | 44.7 | 41.6 | 22.1 |
| Zero | 15.6 | 13.1 | 16.7 |
| Asset (+1 to +10) | 39.8 | 45.2 | 61.2 |

Source: Authors' tabulation of unpublished data from the Survey of Income and Education 1976. Percentages are based on entire handicapped population of the SIE, exclusive of those who lived alone.

Figure B

Relationship Between Family Capacities and Dependent
Person's Needs

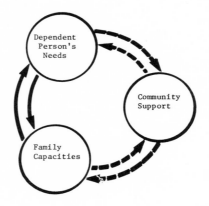

are more likely to have the severely handicapping conditions are
also likely to be part of households where individuals have more
time available to give care. Even holding age constant, however,
the correlation between severity and positive time does not totally
disappear. In Table 9, despite small numbers in the age groups
over 55, in nine out of 14 possible comparisons, the more severely
handicapped showed higher proportions of families with positive
time assets (i.e., higher proportion among the severe than among
the mild; among the severe than among the moderate; and among
the moderate than among the mild).

## Family Income Needs and Outside Sources of Support

If family time capacities somehow adjust to meet the needs of
the disabled person, how then do outside supports from the community become involved in helping disabled individuals and their
families? Showing the connection between individual or family
need and use of outside services would be an ideal test of our
conceptual model. Unfortunately the *Survey of Income and Education* did not treat services; but it did gather detailed information
on income levels and sources of income. These data permit a
description of the two other principal interchanges in our conceptual

model: First, between the disability of the handicapped person and type of outside benefit; and second, between family capacity and sources of outside income.

Overall income figures for our SIE sample, shown in Table 11, reveal stark differences between household income of the handicapped and that of the U.S. population as a whole. Median household income in our unweighted ten percent sample of mildly handicapped is $10,280 compared with a mean of $15,980 for the U.S.

TABLE 11

Median Family Income by Age, Disability Level, and Family Type
of Handicapped Person, SIE 1976

| Age of Handicapped Person | | Disability Level | | | | | |
|---|---|---|---|---|---|---|---|
| | | M i l d | | M o d e r a t e | | S e v e r e | |
| | | Income | Number | Income | Number | Income | Number |
| Under 19 | M-FHH | $15,270 | 569 | $13,273 | 11 | $10,860 | 16 |
| | FHH | 5,935 | 122 | 2,122 | 2 | 6,120 | 5 |
| | MHH | 13,030 | 9 | 750 | 1 | -- | 0 |
| 19-40 | M-FHH | 14,449 | 75 | 12,600 | 203 | 12,159 | 23 |
| | FHH | 5,497 | 17 | 4,300 | 75 | 6,079 | 8 |
| | MHH | 8,475 | 8 | 4,411 | 10 | 13,900 | 1 |
| 41-54 | M-FHH | 15,828 | 79 | 11,673 | 318 | 11,428 | 34 |
| | FHH | 6,470 | 14 | 4,104 | 106 | 3,376 | 11 |
| | MHH | 7,791 | 7 | 3,784 | 33 | 6,120 | 1 |
| 55-64 | M-FHH | 14,668 | 81 | 10,388 | 493 | 8,451 | 37 |
| | FHH | 5,601 | 14 | 2,920 | 140 | 3,398 | 7 |
| | MHH | 6,538 | 5 | 4,900 | 53 | 11,016 | 5 |
| 65-74 | M-FHH | 7,807 | 65 | -- | | 7,857 | 62 |
| | FHH | 3,984 | 27 | -- | | 3,506 | 31 |
| | MHH | 3,500 | 8 | -- | | 5,298 | 1 |
| 75+ | M-FHH | 6,735 | 50 | -- | | 10,896 | 79 |
| | FHH | 3,233 | 39 | -- | | 5,388 | 59 |
| | MHH | 3,392 | 10 | -- | | 5,924 | 17 |
| SIE Median family income | | $10,280 | | $8,707 | | $7,860 | |

U.S. Median family income, 1976:  H.W. families and male-headed families    $16,095

Female-headed families    7,211

Note:  M-FHH  =  Male and female-headed Households.
       FHH    =  Female only headed Households.
       MHH    =  Male only headed Households.

Source:  Authors' tabulation of unpublished data from the Survey of Income and
         Education, 1976.  Based on 5,238 unweighted cases, a 10 percent sample
         of the disabled in the SIE.

in 1977 (calculated from Figure 3.10 of Masnick and Bane, 1980, p. 87). Incomes of the families with moderately and severely handicapped members are even lower. Especially where the handicapped person is an adult, the disability may interfere with employment. In addition more of the severely handicapped are found in the older age groups where household size and retirement also contribute to smaller family income.

Given these facts of life, how do families and communities compensate for the weaker income position of families with handi-

TABLE 12

Percent of Husband-Wife Families Receiving Income by Age, Source and Disability Level of Family Member, SIE 1976

| Age of Handicapped Member | Income Source* | Disability Level | | |
|---|---|---|---|---|
| | | Mild | Moderate | Severe |
| Under 19 | SSI | 4.0 | -- | 12.5 |
| | Social Security | 8.8 | 36.4 | -- |
| | AFDC | 7.4 | 9.1 | 18.8 |
| Ages 19-40 | SSI | 1.2 | 10.8 | 26.1 |
| | Social Security | 7.8 | 19.7 | 34.8 |
| | AFDC | 4.1 | 11.3 | 13.0 |
| | Public Assistance | 1.0 | 3.9 | 4.3 |
| | Retirement | 3.7 | 6.9 | 17.4 |
| Ages 41-54 | SSI | 1.6 | 10.4 | 8.8 |
| | Social Security | 9.0 | 27.7 | 61.8 |
| | Retirement | 4.8 | 11.0 | 20.6 |
| | Pension | 1.1 | 6.0 | 17.6 |
| | VA | 12.5 | 14.5 | 26.5 |
| Ages 55-64 | SSI | 3.4 | 9.1 | 13.5 |
| | Social Security | 27.7 | 57.8 | 67.6 |
| | AFDC | .7 | 2.0 | 8.1 |
| | Pension | 7.5 | 16.2 | 18.9 |
| 65 and over | SSI | 8.8 | | 17.0 |
| | Public Assistance | 1.4 | | 3.5 |
| | VA | 7.6 | | 9.9 |

* Only those income sources (other than wages, salary and self-employment) are listed under each age group which exhibited a significant difference in the percentage of mildly, moderately or severely dependent who received them. "Public assistance" refers to programs other than AFDC.

Source: Authors' tabulation of unpublished data from the Survey of Income and Education, 1976. Based on 5,238 unweighted cases, a 10 percent sample of the dependent persons in the SIE.

Figure C
Model of the Relationship Between Dependent Person's
Needs and Community Supports

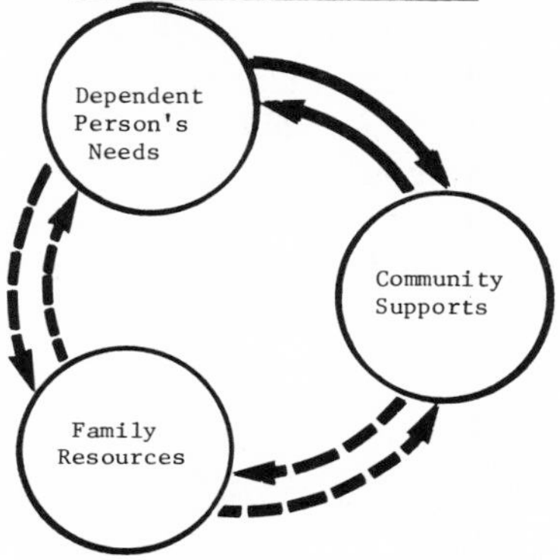

capped members? First, it appears that families have greater access to certain entitlements and sources of outside income, the greater the disability of their handicapped member. Table 12 shows the proportions of Husband-Wife families with a handicapped member who receive outside income from Supplemental Security Income payments (SSI), Social Security, Aid to Families with Dependent Children (AFDC), Public Assistance, retirement, private pensions, and Veterans Assistance (VA). Eight categories of such income were noted.

More families with a severely or moderately handicapped member received all these types of income than did families of the mildly handicapped. The types of income where a clear trend emerged in favor of the more disabled were associated with certain age groups and not others. For example, in three age groups, under 19, 19-40, and 55-64, more families of the severely handicapped and moderately handicapped received SSI, Social Security, and AFDC than did the mildly handicapped. Such a pattern was not evident with respect to AFDC in the 41-54 or over 65 age groups. Nor did the pattern hold for Social Security in the over 65 age group. Yet overall one concludes nevertheless that more families received financial support, the more disabled their handicapped member. This appears to be one type of confirmation of our conceptual model related to the interchange between outside support and disability of the handicapped member as shown in Figure C.

Finally, we turn to the third interchange—between family capacities and outside support. To test this concept we need to hold constant age and level of severity of the handicapped member and ask how support varies by family structure. Do female-headed families get more outside help than husband-wife families, for example? Our data as shown in Table 13 provide overwhelming evidence that they do. Taking just the middle-age groups, five types of assistance are more frequently found among female-headed than husband-wife families: Supplemental Security Income, Social Se-

TABLE 13

Percent of Husband-Wife Families and Female-Headed Families
with Handicapped Member ages 41-54 Who Are Receiving
Outside Income by Disability Level of Family
Member and Source of Income, SIE 1976

| Income Source* (Recipients ages 41-54) | Disability Level | Family Type** | |
|---|---|---|---|
| | | M-FHH | FHH |
| Public Assistance | Mild | 0.3 | 3.1 |
| | Moderate | 3.5 | 12.3 |
| | Severe | -- | 18.2 |
| SSI | Mild | 1.6 | 3.1 |
| | Moderate | 10.4 | 31.1 |
| | Severe | 8.8 | 54.5 |
| Social Security | Mild | 9.0 | 35.4 |
| | Moderate | 27.7 | 41.5 |
| | Severe | 61.8 | 54.5 |
| AFDC | Mild | 1.3 | 7.7 |
| | Moderate | 6.3 | 28.3 |
| | Severe | 2.9 | 9.1 |
| Alimony | Mild | 0.3 | 13.8 |
| | Moderate | 0.3 | 4.7 |
| | Severe | -- | 9.1 |

  * Retirement, Pension, and VA do not appear on this table because no clear
    trend emerged that was associated with family type.

 ** M-FHH  = Male-female headed families
    FHH    = Female-headed families

Source:  Author's tabulation of unpublished data from the Survey of Income and
         Education, 1976. Based on 5,238 unweighted cases, a 10 percent sample
         of the dependent persons in the SIE.

Figure D

Model of the Relationship Between Family
Capacity and Community Support

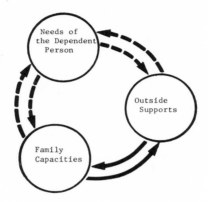

curity, AFDC, Public Assistance, and alimony. In addition the differences generally hold across all severity levels.

These findings on differences in outside support that are associated with family structure confirm the third interchange in our conceptual model as shown in Figure D. Structural factors (such as female-headedness) are related to the receipt of outside support.

Our analysis of the SIE data provides evidence, though somewhat limited and impressionistic, of family adjustments and impacts anticipated in our conceptual framework. Care-giving families are both poorer and smaller than families in the general population; perhaps these differences characterize the "survivors" among families who assume these responsibilities for dependent and disabled relatives. The data point to adjustments in family time and to the outside supports that reach these families from public programs.

The analysis suggests, moreover, that on both micro and macro levels the relationships among the dependent person, the family, and community resources are delicately balanced. This is true, for example, of the special burdens in care-giving families headed by females and in families with young children.

Much research, particularly of a longitudinal nature, is needed to study the outcomes and the processes of family home care. This exploration has raised some key issues that such research should address.

# NOTES

1. Moroney discusses definitions at the beginning of his paper in Part III. Barry offers these definitions: Residual limitation resulting from a congenital defect, disease, or injury has been termed an *impairment*; this can be alleviated or remediated through devices or medical care. A *disability* is an inability to perform some key life functions; this can be remediated through training, or devices or medical care. When a disability interacts with the environment to impose impediments to the individual's goals for travel or work, for example, the individual has a *handicap*. Handicapping conditions can be remediated through changes in the environment, or training of the individual, or both (Barry, 1975, p. 4).

2. Moroney, in his paper in this collection, puts the number of handicapped people at 3.7 million. "Handicap" refers to the disadvantage due to the loss or reduction of functional ability. And while "handicap" is not a precise indicator of the need for personal care, Moroney observes that this group of almost four million "will make demands on families, possibly heighten stress on family life, and at a minimum, force families with handicapped members to function differently than most families." Based on the need for "ordinary personal care," DeJong estimates that there are 3.5 million Americans in this situation, excluding those below working age (DeJong 1978, pp. 3-5). Neither estimate, however, clearly distinguishes between people living in institutions, living alone, or with family.

Callahan and his colleagues concluded that between 60 and 85 percent of all disabled or impaired people are helped by the family in a significant way (Callahan et al., p. 2). Another estimate placed the number of people in Massachusetts in 1975 not in institutions who needed help with personal care from someone else, either regularly or irregularly, at 2.9 percent of the population (DeJong, 1977, p. 3). Applying this percentage to the total United States population in 1970, the latest year for which the number of noninstitutionalized persons is known, produces a national population of 5.8 million in need of personal care.

3. The second type of comparison could be done by examining characteristics of next-of-kin in the *Survey of Institutionalized Persons* (U.S. Bureau of the Census, 1978). Some of this analysis has already been done for the frail elderly living in institutions as compared with those living in the community. See Soldo and Sharma, 1980.

4. As is evident in tables 8, 9, and 11, these definitions resulted in no moderately dependent people in the older age groups because that definition relied on school and work questions that were not asked of persons over 65.

# REFERENCES

Barrett, Nancy Smith. 1979. "Data Needs for Evaluating the Labor Market Status of Women." In B.B. Reagan (ed.), *Issues in Federal Statistical Needs Relating to Women*. U.S. Department of Commerce, Bureau of the Census, Current Population Reports, Special Studies Series P-23, No. 83.

Barry, Patricia. 1975. "Summary of the Comprehensive Needs Study," Working Paper 0981-04, The Urban Institute.

Berkowitz, Monroe, William G. Johnson and Edward H. Murphy. 1976. *Public Policy Toward Disability*, New York: Prager Publishers.

Blenkner, Margaret. 1963. "Social Work and Family Relationships in Later Life." In E. Shanas and G. Streib (eds.), *Social Structure and the Family: Generational Relationships*. Englewood Cliffs, N.J.: Prentice-Hall.

Boggs, Elizabeth M. and R. Lee Henney. (undated.) "A Numerical and Functional Description of the Developmental Disabilities Population," (for Non-Institutionalized Individuals), EMC Institute, produced under Developmental Disabilities Project of National Significance #54-P-71220/3-02, DHEW.

Brody, E.M. 1978. "The Aging of the Family." *Annals of the American Academy of Political and Social Science* 438 (July): 13-27.

Brody, Stanley J., S.W. Poulshock, and C.F. Masciocchi. 1978. "The Family Caring Unit: A Major Consideration in the Long-Term Support System." *The Gerontologist* 18 (6): 556-561.

Brownstein, Elise and Helen G. Berkley. "Medical Social Work Home Intervention Project." Boston: The Children's Hospital Medical Center, 1979, unpublished.

Callahan, James J., Jr., Lawrence D. Diamond, Janet Z. Giele, and Robert Morris. "Responsibilities of Families for their Severely Disabled Elders." *Health Care Financing Review*, 1980, 1(3): 29-48.

Congressional Budget Office. 1977. *Health Differentials Between White and Nonwhite Americans*. Washington, D.C.: USGPO.

DeJong, Gerben. 1977. "The Need for Personal Care Services by Severely Physically Disabled Citizens of Massachusetts." The Levinson Policy Institute, Waltham MA: Brandeis University.

_____. 1978. "Disability, Home Care, and Relative Responsibility: A Legal Perspective." Boston: Medical Rehabilitation Institute, Tufts-New England Medical Center.

Giele, Janet Zollinger. 1978. *Women and the Future: Changing Sex Roles in Modern America*. New York: Free Press.

Giele, Janet Zollinger. 1981. "A Review of Selected Data Sources on the Family's Role in Long-Term Care." Waltham, Mass.: Brandeis University, Levinson Policy Institute.

Kobrin, Frances E. 1976. "The Primary Individual and the Family: Changes in Living Arrangements in the United States Since 1940." *Journal of Marriage and the Family* 38 (May): 233-239.

Maddox, George L. 1975. "Families as Context and Resource in Chronic Illness." In Sylvia Sherwood (ed.), *Long-Term Care*. New York: Spectrum Publications.

Mahoney, Kevin J. 1977. "A National Perspective on Community Differences in the Interaction of the Aged with Their Adult Children." Madison, Wisc.: University of Wisconsin–Madison, Fay McBeath Institute.

Masnick, George, and Mary Jo Bane. 1980. *The Nation's Families, 1960-1990*. Boston: Auburn House.

Moroney, Robert M. 1976. *The Family and the State: Considerations for Social Policy*. London: Longmans.

Morell, Bonnie Brown. 1979. "Deinstitutionalization: Those Left Behind." *Social Work*, November 1979, pp. 528-532.

Morris, Robert and Paul Youket. 1980. "Major Options in Long-Term Care—Background and Framework," in Stanley S. Wallack and James J. Callahan, Jr. *Major Reforms in Long-Term Care: A Systematic Comparison of the Options*. Waltham, Mass.: Center for Health Policy Analysis and Research, Brandeis University.

National Center for Health Statistics (NCHS). 1969. "Marital Status and Living Arrangements before Admission to Nursing and Personal Care Homes, United States, May-June 1964." *Vital and Health Statistics*. Series 12, No. 12. Washington, D.C.

National Center for Health Statistics (NCHS). 1973. "Characteristics of Residents in Nursing and Personal Care Homes, United States, June-August 1969." *Vital and Health Statistics*. Series 12, No. 19. Rockville, Maryland.

Perlman, Robert and Roland L. Warren. 1977. *Families in the Energy Crisis*. Cambridge, Mass.: Ballinger.

Rosenmayr, Leopold. 1977. "The Family—A Source of Hope for the Elderly?" In E. Shanas and M.B. Sussman (eds.), *Family, Bureaucracy, and the Elderly*. Durham, N.C.: Duke University Press.

Schorr, Alvin L. 1980. *Thy Father and Thy Mother: A Second Look at Filial Responsibility and Family Policy*. Washington, D.C.: U.S. Department of Health and Human Services, Social Security Administration. July.

Siegel, Jacob S., Mark D. Herrenbruck, Donald S. Akers, and Jeffrey S. Passel. 1978. "Demographic Aspects of Aging and the Older Population in the United States." *Current*

*Population Reports: Special Studies*. Series P-23, No. 59. Washington, D.C.: USGPO.

Silverstone, Barbara. 1978. "An Overview of Research on Informal Supports: Implications for Policy and Practice." Paper presented at the Annual Meeting of the Gerontological Society, Dallas, November 17.

Soldo, Beth J., and Mahesh Sharma. 1980. "Families Who Purchase vs. Families Who Provide Care Services to Elderly Relatives." Paper presented at the Annual Meeting of the Gerontological Society of Amercia, November 22-26, San Diego, California.

*Statistical Abstract of the United States*. 1976.

Townsend, Peter. 1957. *The Family Life of Old People: An Inquiry in East London*. London: Routledge and Kegan Paul.

Treas, Judith. 1975. "Aging and the Family." In D.S. Woodruff and J.E. Birren (eds.), *Aging: Scientific Perspectives and Social Issues*. New York: Van Nostrand.

U.S. Bureau of the Census. 1976. Raw data on tape. *Survey of Income and Education*.

U.S. Bureau of the Census. 1975. *Current Population Reports*. Series P-25, No. 614, "Estimates of the Population of the United States by Age, Sex, and Race: 1970 to 1975," U.S. Government Printing Office.

_____. 1976. *Current Population Reports*. Series P-60, No. 101, "Money Income in 1974 of Families and Persons in the United States," U.S. Government Printing Office.

_____. 1976. *Current Population Reports*. Series P-20, No. 292, "Population Profile of the United States: 1975," U.S. Government Printing Office.

_____. 1978. *Current Population Reports*. Special Studies, Series P-23, No. 69, "1976 Survey of Institutionalized Persons."

U.S. Senate. 1971. "The Multiple Hazards of Age and Race: The Situation of Aged Blacks in the United States." A working paper. Special Committee on Aging. Washington, D.C.: U.S. Government Printing Office.

# PART II: DEMANDS AND RESOURCES

# Introduction to Part II

The six papers in this part of the collection examine the dynamics and the outcomes of home care, particularly as they affect the families involved. While the writers deal with different populations (developmentally disabled children, unmarried adolescent mothers, the frail elderly, and the mental patient), and while they express quite disparate views as to what is "the problem," they all grapple with these questions: How can the welfare of the dependent person be protected? How can families cope? What social interventions are desirable and, in terms of cost, feasible?

Most of the writers, implicitly or explicitly, tie these questions together in a conceptualization—similar to that in the previous chapter—in which the outcomes of home care depend on the interaction between the demands presented by the dependent person's condition and the resources the family brings, sometimes augmented by community agencies. These outcomes range at one end of a spectrum from good care, family well-being, and reasonable cost, to inadequate care, family breakdown, and unnecessary, costly institutionalization, at the opposite end. All this is seen as a process extending over time, which itself alters the demands, the resources, and the outcomes.

Some demands on family resources are concrete and immediate in their impact, such as incursions on the time and energies of family members and on their finances. This is apparent from the following account:

Fatigue appears to be a way of life for many parents of handicapped children. Some of the children require almost 24 hour nursing care. With other children there may be physical fatigue of parents caused by heavy lifting, bathing, dressing and frequent visits for medical care and educational problems. Chronic low back pain is a frequent cause of complaint from mothers of heavy children with c.p. . . . (There) also may be unpredictable emergency visits to the hospital in the middle of the night; like those of sudden midnight episodes of croup in mongoloid. Upper respiratory infection often keeps parents awake; physical fatigue is augmented by lack of sleep. (Howell, 1973, quoted in Gordon, 1980, p. 34)

Potentially there are many serious effects that flow from the presence of a dependent person in the home and the family's response—tension, stigma, social isolation, plans and hopes frustrated, etc. We refer to these as potential burdens because families differ considerably as to whether, how much, and why they experience caring for a relative as burdensome or noxious or rewarding.

Some families will not undertake the caring responsibility at all, while others are like the grandmother quoted in the Klerman paper (below) who said of her unmarried daughter and her new grandchild: "After all, fifteen is kind of young to marry, and we wanted her to finish high school and go to college. Anyway, I've had ten kids, so as long as I can remember there's always been a baby in the house, and this one is our pride and joy." Why does this woman find joy while her neighbor down the street, faced with the same situation, feels only shame, drudgery, and resentment?

There are, roughly speaking, three kinds of explanations in the literature for the differences among families in their coping performance and in the impacts they experience:

(a) *psychological* variations among caregivers.
(b) *socially conditioned* responses that vary, for example, by ethnic and religious groups, social class etc.
(c) *situational* differences such as the physical and emotional state of the dependent person; the stage in the family's life cycle; the use of supportive services, etc.

Our task here is to review the findings concerning the impacts of home care on families and to explore the alternative (or complementary) explanations for the quite different ways in which families perceive their situation and respond to it.

The term "family burden" conveys the stresses and strains that home care can produce. These are highly interrelated and in the discussion that follows no order of importance is implied. Family members expend time and energy on the routines that constitute much of living together—shopping, food preparation, eating, house cleaning—and renew their energies through sleep, rest, and recreation. The presence of a dependent person impinges on these activities. The hours and the physical and emotional energy that care of a dependent relative requires, e.g., dressing, feeding, doing mountains of laundry, must be diverted from other activities or from rest.

The dimension of time *per se* was used in a study of care of the elderly at home (Gurland, 1978). "Personal time dependency" was defined as time spent "providing services in direct contact with the dependent where the withholding of the service would seriously threaten the dependent's continued existence in that setting"; i.e., services above and beyond those we are all accustomed to receive as part of the exchange of social life. Gurland and his associates found that "perceived inconvenience" was the most significant factor in bringing a family to the point of institutionalizing an older relative and that the *amount of time* spent in caring was the factor which best explained inconvenience.

The prolonged disruption of household routines and the demands on the family's time and energy can place the physical and mental health of the non-disabled members in jeopardy. The occurrence of "burn-out" or physical and mental exhaustion is not uncommon. A Social Security Administration study of the impact of disability on the family concludes with this comment: "Chronic poor health impoverished not only those it afflicted, but also those living with them" (Franklin, 1977). Gurland reported that serious depression was found in one-fourth of the families with whom dependent elderly people lived in New York City. An important point, which reappears in the discussion of policy options in Part III of this collection, is made by Horejsi (below) who objects strenuously to the irrationality of our present policies which require many families almost to destroy themselves before the community offers services that might well have forestalled such an outcome.

There is no evidence that relatives living elsewhere or friends and neighbors make a significant contribution to helping with the extra work and other burdens involved in home care. Franklin, for example, found that most families received very little household help from relatives outside the immediate family. The same was true of financial assistance.

Little research has been done on the financial costs of maintaining a dependent relative at home—the expenses for special equipment, food, or medicine; the hiring of sitters; renovations in the family's dwelling; earnings foregone; extra expenses for traveling, when that is possible; and other out-of-pocket expenditures. The dollar value of services provided by families and friends of impaired elderly people was estimated in a study in Cleveland to be about $200 per month (Comptroller General, 1977). Further research is needed and two variables will be particularly important in this connection—one is the nature of the dependent person's condition and the kinds of services and equipment that are required, and the other is the extent to which outside resources, in cash or in kind, are utilized to cushion the direct costs for the family.

Prager, analyzing data collected by Sussman, found an attitude that suggests that financial concerns are not paramount. In 88 percent of the households surveyed "financial considerations were *not* given as the reason for the family's need to turn to community or governmental resources when burdened with the care of a chronically ill aged relative." The majority of those interviewed said that they could manage the financial burden if the community would provide the supportive services required by their disabled relatives (Prager, 1977). However, financial cost emerged as a "major stress" in a study of families with retarded children. Apart from extra medical costs, the expenses entailed in "maintaining normal family functioning" were the most frequently noted adverse effect of home care (Aldrich et al., 1971 cited in Morell, below).

It is not clear under what circumstances the presence of a disabled person has the effect of lowering a family's total income through a loss of earnings on the part of the dependent relative and/or on the part of non-disabled members of the family who are restricted in their labor force participation because they are care-providers. Franklin notes that the earnings of husbands and wives of disabled spouses are lower than the general level, but what factors account for this difference remain to be studied (Franklin *op. cit.*, pp. 9-10).

These have been generalizations about the burdens of home care but families vary greatly in how they perceive and experience the adjustments required by these responsibilities. However "objective" time and money seem, for example, re-allocating them within a family will generate different reactions from family to family. One interpretation of this, which rests primarily on *psychological factors*, is set forth in this report on 303 families with very severely disabled children with a variety of disabilities:

> The researchers found that although the degree of stress experienced by the mother was partly due to features of her environment (financial resources, whether she was able to work outside the home if she so wished, the amount of help and support received from relatives and friends, the child's health, whether the child played normally and whether he was normally active), these factors were not by themselves enough to explain why some mothers experienced comparatively little stress and others a great deal. They suggest an alternative hypothesis, that the level of stress is determined by internal factors—by the physiology and personality of the mother—and that these internal factors are not affected in any specific way by the external social and physical conditions of the family and the child. (Bradshaw and Lawton, 1978, summarized in Gordon, 1980, p. 38)

But before we can consider individual variability due to psychological factors, we must deal with another generalization, namely, that it is "natural" for family members to give intimate, physical help to each other. This capacity to feel compassion and behave lovingly toward the weak and the dependent, a psychoanalyst argues, is in great part determined by the lessons each of us learned during our prenatal and postnatal dependency, "that miserable, extended, helpless state in which we are born and remain for so long" (Gaylin, 1978, pp. 3-5). The foundation for becoming a caring human being rests on the infant's "fused image of security and food" and sense of being loved.

The further claim is made from a psychosocial perspective that the emotional effects of family care are beneficial and highly desirable. Klerman (below) for instance, makes this point in terms of the healthy development of the babies of teenage mothers—and the mothers themselves—as they experience love and support through daily contact with grandparents and other relatives.

The view that the caring impulse runs deep in human beings is not universally accepted. Morris (below) writes that "we simply do not know whether the dynamics of family relationships are

governed by a basic, fundamental desire" to care for each other or
by a tendency to divest the family of responsibility for members
who are vulnerable and dependent. Depending on our understanding of this, he points out, our public policies can either reinforce
a basic dynamic in families or they can attempt to influence behavior away from the normative standard in the direction that
society favors.

Alvin Schorr attests to the vast extent of caring that does exist:
"Family mutual support may constitute the deepest well of altruism
in the Nation" (Schorr, 1980). But the very bio-psychosocial processes that may generate this altruism can also lead in the opposite direction, toward an avoidance of the caring role. Gaylin
believes the outcome will depend on the nature of the early caretaker and the nature of the child. Thus, a mother "may not respond
with the same intuitive caring to a crippled or deformed child as
she would to a healthy one. She may be so threatened, guilty, or
simply repelled that those caring attitudes that intuitively are designed to insure the survival of the species will not be elicited"
(Gaylin, pp. 26-29).

It is not clear how deep or shallow, how widespread or how
limited, is the altruism that undergirds family home care. What is
clearer is that families (and the individuals within them) differ substantially in their motivation to undertake home care and in their
capacity to sustain it. One can reasonably presume, moreover, that
these variations are also reflected in the various ways in which
families experience the consequences of this undertaking. Take,
for example, the impact on relationships within the family. In some
situations, marital stability as well as parent-child and inter-sibling
relationships deteriorate under the weight of prolonged tension and
disruption of living patterns. Franklin notes in the research cited
above that more marriages end in divorce or separation for disabled
people than for the non-disabled.

But in other situations, there are positive or neutral effects on
family life. Gordon reports that the general trend of research on
marital relationships in families with a handicapped child suggests
that the impact will depend on the relationship that existed prior
to the birth of the child. A sound, established relationship can
survive or even be strengthened by the experience of providing
care at home; a relationship of short duration or a shaky one can
be shattered (Gordon, 1980, p. 42).

Much of the writing in this area focuses on the whole family as a social system that is subject to stress from changes in its environment. The "stress model" of how families function in the face of crises depicts the family as a system of complementary roles. When its equilibrium is disturbed, as occurs when one person takes on the "sick role," compensatory adjustments are made in other roles so that the family can return to homeostasis (Wawzonek, 1974). If this does not happen the family becomes disorganized, according to this theory, and cannot function adequately.

Lorenz does not find the stress model so useful for illuminating the dynamics of family home care.* The model assumes that a family will either absorb the stress or utterly succumb to it, but does not specify how families can and do solve problems in the face of stress. Moreover, it conceptualizes the family as a homeostatic structure whose primary goal is to resist change and maintain a stable equilibrium. Lorenz proposes an alternative model that would view the family as a cognitive, information-processing, problem-solving system capable of actively exploiting opportunities in its environment, such as community services or informal support networks.

The stress model is helpful, however, precisely because it calls attention to the nature and the sources of stress and to the useful concept of role and role strain. Monk (below) refers to the role conflicts that are bound to occur when filial obligations impinge on the husband-wife relationship, one example of strain resulting from "concurrent demands on beleaguered individuals with multiple roles to fill." Some information is available on the roles in the family that are most affected by the responsibilities of home care. A study in Massachusetts found that the person who most frequently helps with personal care was the spouse in 37 percent of the cases studied or a parent in 34 percent (DeJong, 1977, p. 27).

In Gurland's research on the elderly, the "key support" was the spouse in half the cases and a child in one-third of the cases, most often a daughter or daughter-in-law. Gurland's finding is one indication that the role strains that occur in home care often affect women of working age, the traditional sources of care for the sick and infirm. Franklin remarks that "the wives of disabled men indicated that their increased labor force participation came as a response to illness rather than other factors . . . such women appear

---

*I am indebted to Kenneth A. Lorenz, M.D. for this discussion of family models and family burdens, which was developed in an unpublished paper written at the Florence Heller Graduate School for Advanced Studies in Social Welfare, Brandeis University, 1978.

to have shifted their role to offset the economic loss caused by illness" (Franklin, 1977, p. 9).

The causes of stress in families with handicapped children were studied by Bradshaw and Lawton, who found that the level of stress varied among women according to "their satisfaction or dissatisfaction with their roles as housewife or worker"; whether they got out of the house as much as they wanted to, and whether the family had had a vacation within the last year. They found no association between stress and size of family, though other studies have found such a connection (Gordon, 1980). Strains were found by Bradshaw and Lawton and other researchers where parents felt embarrassment or stigma as a result of having a retarded child.

Differences among families in terms of their ability to manage home care also stem from each family's history and experience. For example, the strengths or limitations that are left following other crises differ from family to family. The present size and composition of a family, its income, its negotiating skills in the maze-like market of community services, its other problems—all these play a part in shaping the response and the impact that families experience, even when the condition and needs of the dependent persons are roughly similar.

Stress and frustration on the one hand and high motivation and successful coping on the other hand are attributed by some writers, as we have seen, to psychological and physiological variations among individuals and families. Another line of explanation of the differences in coping and in impact looks to the larger social system as the source of people's norms and expectations—and therefore of their frustrations or successes. Social class, ethnicity, and religion are associated with different ways in which families perceive and evaluate their situation and then react to it. Demos, in Part III of this collection, traces changes that have occurred in this respect in the course of the past 300 years of American history.

Farber is a principal articulator of this approach. As one of the first researchers in this area, his work with the families of mentally retarded children early turned to the social environment to understand what meaning the family gave to its situation. "Larger social forces," he says in his paper in this collection, "seem to mold the person's view of how the world operates and of the interpretation of disappointing or noxious events." Thus, for instance, he has found that the higher the socioeconomic status of a family, the greater the negative impact of labeling a child retarded.

Farber rejects what he considers a "medical model" or deficiency model of developmentally delayed children and their families; he believes that it leads to "blaming the victim" when a family fails to cope with its problems. Farber argues that the motivation and capability of a family are influenced by religious beliefs, education, the existence of supportive kin and friends, and the like. While he focuses primarily on developmentally disabled children, Farber speaks to the broad issues that cut across home care of many kinds of disabled family members. In a sober vein, he insists that disappointment, pain, and tragedy are unavoidable and normal, however much they do not fit with the aspirations and illusions of the American dream of finding solutions to all problems through technology and achieving "success" in all endeavors.

The objection might be raised here that a family's adjustment to the birth and the care of a handicapped child is not comparable to the situation of an older woman suddenly called upon to provide daily care to a disabled husband. A considerable literature, for example, deals with the very specific psychological and emotional problems faced by mothers and fathers of retarded children. Doubtless certain of their difficulties are different in kind from some of the problems of the elderly couple. But it can also be argued that there is a large area of overlap that has to do with a person's motivation to take on the responsibilities of home care often at considerable personal cost. These attitudes, it can be argued, are incorporated in each of us from that part of the socioeconomic system in which we were socialized—as middle-class Protestants, or low income Blacks, or Orthodox Jews, etc. In this sense, the capacity for providing care is heavily influenced by cultural and social determinants.

A third approach to understanding what makes home care viable or insupportable rests on a situational analysis. This is expressed in several elements in Horejsi's model, presented in the next paper, in which he emphasizes the interaction among these factors: (1) the family's motivation to solve or cope with the problem, (2) their physical, emotional, and intellectual capacities, (3) *the seriousness of the problem and the difficulty of the task facing the family,* and (4) *such factors of opportunity as formal and informal resources in their immediate environment.* Using this situational analysis, he explores the results of increases and decreases in these factors in order to have a basis for predicting when a family will cope adequately and when the dependent person's need will be appropriately satisfied.

The variations in "the seriousness of the problem" facing different families are tremendous. True, this is in part a matter of subjective judgment by each family, but it is also a matter of stark, objective differences in the dependent person's ability to get in and out of bed alone, to eat without being fed, to associate with friends of the family who visit, etc. And these gradations make family care more or less likely, more or less manageable. To give only one illustration of an almost infinite number, Segal (below) points out that willingness of families to accept a discharged mental patient back in their homes is influenced by the duration of their relative's stay in mental hospital and by the severity of the patient's symptoms.

So too with the "formal and informal resources in their immediate environment." The viability of home care can hinge, under certain circumstances, on the amount and quality of supportive assistance the family can add to its own resources of time, energy, money, and the like. A majority of the 400 families questioned in a survey in Alabama concerning the impact of a disabled child did not believe "the disabled person had a negative effect on other family members," but they "did indicate quite strongly the need for assistance. . . . When the handicapped person was seen as having affected the family, it was more often in the areas such as trips, vacations, visiting, shopping, or going to movies or to church, or whether the mother will work. The results also showed that time demands, physical demands, and money problems were more often indicated as important" (Dunlap and Hollingsworth, 1977).

The significant point about the situational approach to home care is that it brings into consideration interventions from outside the family. Unlike the psychological factors and the broad social forces that contribute to shaping a family's response to home care, the situational elements are subject to deliberate manipulation through policy and administrative decisions. This aspect of family home care is the subject of Part III of the book.

What we have said in this introduction is that there can be heavy burdens on families who undertake home care, burdens that have serious implications for the dependent person's well-being and for the physical, emotional, and financial health of the rest of the family. To what extent people come to this challenge with a "caring impulse" derived from their childhood experiences is a moot point. We have established that there is a wide variation among families in their willingness to take on home care and in the effects it has on them.

Three ways of explaining these variations—the psychological, the social, and the situational—have been summarized. The information and analysis contained in the papers that follow these comments will make it quite clear that there is no exclusivity or priority among the three explanatory positions. As is often the case with complex human processes, family home care can be best understood as the resultant of all three kinds of influence interacting with each other and with the lives, thoughts, and feelings of the people involved.

# Social and Psychological Factors in Family Care

## Charles R. Horejsi

Not many years ago, there were only two options available to developmentally disabled individuals and their families. The handicapped person could either remain with his family or enter an institution. With the first option, the family and the handicapped individual were more or less on their own; there were few community resources from which to draw support and assistance. They struggled with their problems and coped as best they could. If individuals were to be admitted to large multi-purpose institutions, they would have access to some special services, but institutional environments left much to be desired. The longer they were to remain, the less likely they would ever return to their family and the less able they would be to function outside of the institution.

Gradually, a third option developed; namely, the network of programs we term community-based services. This new system of community-based services now stood between the family and the institution. Fewer persons went into institutions and some left the institutions and entered community programs. Of interest, however, is the fact that the flow of handicapped persons out of the family continued. Instead of going from family to institution, handicapped persons moved from home into community residential programs. Few of those leaving the institutions returned to their families.

It is my understanding that this conference hopes to take a closer look at family care as an alternative to both community residential programs and institutions. An examination of family care must grapple with many complex questions. Is family care a viable option? If it is, for what kinds of families, for persons with what types of handicaps, and under what circumstances? Is it, for ex-

Source: Horejsi, Charles R. "Social and Psychological Factors in Family Care." In *Family Care of Developmentally Disabled Members: Conference Proceedings,* edited by Robert H. Bruininks and Gordon C. Krantz. University of Minnesota, 1979. Reprinted with permission.

ample, workable in two-parent families but not in single-parent families or in families where both parents work outside the home? If it is an option for some families, for what length of time is it workable? Are there stages in the family life cycle when it is an option and stages where it is unworkable? Is it possibly an option in situations where the handicapped person has never left home, but unworkable once the disabled person has left home and spent time in either a community group home or an institution? Can the ordinary family with all of its ordinary problems and concerns adequately deal with the extraordinary problems and concerns presented by a severely handicapped family member? Finally, do existing service programs and public policies encourage or discourage family care? I doubt that we will have all the answers at the end of this two-day conference. However, if we can identify the key questions and sharpen the issues, our time will have been well spent.

## *WHY FAMILY CARE?*

We may begin our exploration with the question, "Why family care?" All across the human services, there is a renewed interest in home-based services. Home health care is an excellent example. Sussman (1977) has noted that . . . as services and the population increase, skyrocketing costs for services threaten the society's economy and its ability to maintain existing services or to provide new services . . . Consequently, there is interest in alternative, less costly systems for meeting the needs of dependent populations.

> One approach is to examine the extent to which family networks might be able to provide such care, particularly if resources are made available (p. 367).

While it is clear that some of the reasons behind the new interest in family care are economic, and hence political, there are also sound professional reasons for taking a second look at the family as a basic resource for persons with special needs. Skarnulis (1976a) has noted that:

> The most effective deinstitutionalization program possible is the one that prevents removal of mentally retarded persons from their home in the first place. Most children are not

"placed" by their parents but are "taken" from the homes of parents because no alternatives are available (to help the parents cope) (p. 63).

If we can assume that family care is desirable, why do so many handicapped persons leave their homes before the normal age of emancipation? What are the social and psychological forces that "push" or "pull" the handicapped person out of his own home? If we can identify those factors, especially the ones over which we can exert some control, we will be in a better position to provide added incentives for family care.

## DEFINITION OF FAMILY CARE

Before going further I want to explain how I am using the term family care, at least for the purposes of this paper. Obviously, family care exists when a handicapped member lives with his natural family—either parents, siblings or other relatives. However, I see two types of family care: (1) habilitative family care and (2) ordinary family care. By habilitative family care I am referring to the care, training and supervision of a developmentally disabled person, within the context of his own family, wherein adult family members assume major responsibility for ordinary parenting, socialization, day-to-day personal care and some responsibility for the implementation of individual habilitation plans. Thus, habilitative family care is planned and occurs in conjunction with other support and habilitation services.

In contrast, I apply the term ordinary family care to those situations in which a handicapped individual remains with his family but does not receive appropriate habilitation services. Prior to the development of community-based services, most family care was of this type. Unfortunately, there are still many cases of ordinary family care; the developmentally disabled individual lives with his family but does not receive the special services needed. The handicapped individual receives food and shelter and the concern of family members but this care is not supplemented by professional services such as those provided for in P. L. 94-103.

## THE M-C-O FRAMEWORK

As a way of sorting out factors affecting family care, I have used the simple framework called the Motivation, Capacity and Opportunity Framework. This construct suggests that the ability of an individual or family to deal successfully with a task or problem is a function of:

1. The *seriousness of that problem* or difficulty of task,
2. Their *motivation* to solve or cope with the problem,
3. Their *capacity* (physical, emotional, intellectual, etc.), and
4. Factors of *opportunity* (i.e., formal and informal resources in their immediate environment and wider social and economic forces).

When the M-C-O Framework is applied to the family of a developmentally disabled child, for example, we would say that the family's ability to provide family care is a function of (1) the seriousness and complexity of the problems presented by the child's condition, (2) each family member's motivation, (3) their capacity, and (4) resources and restrictions in their environment. This framework can be presented as a simple formula in which:

FC = ability to provide family care
M  = motivation
C  = capacity
O  = environmental opportunity
P  = problems, needs, demands of developmentally disabled family member.

Thus:

$$FC = \frac{M \times C \times O}{P}$$

In case you have forgotten your algebra, please do not be frightened by this mathematical-like formula. It is simply a framework to which we can attach some ideas about family care. We can play around with this formula and make a few important points. Note that the formula indicates that in order to elevate or enhance (#) the family's ability to provide family care, we must find a way of increasing (#) their motivation or their capacity or the opportunity of their environment. This is shown below.

$$FC\# = \frac{M\# \times C\# \times O\#}{P}$$

The services and supports that increase motivation, capacity and opportunity can be symbolized by (S). Thus, we have

$$FC = \frac{(M \times C \times O)\, S}{P}$$

Most of us associated with programs for developmentally disabled persons are in the business of providing the (S) in the formula. One other important point is illustrated by this little formula. As (P) becomes larger, the ability to provide family care increases.

$$FC\# = \frac{MCO}{P\#}$$

To go one step further, if you want to maintain the family's ability to provide care while the child's problem becomes more serious (P#), you must provide more and more services (S#) in order to sustain their motivation, increase their capacity and/or expand environmental opportunity for family care. One final point can be made. No amount of services can compensate for a complete lack of motivation, capacity and opportunity. Moreover, even if a family has motivation and capacity, no amount of services can compensate for powerful social and economic forces that severely restrict opportunity.

## *MOTIVATION*

Motivation can be viewed as a balance between the "pull" of hope and the "push" of discomfort. We are drawn toward that which we value and we push away from that which creates discomfort. We can tolerate discomfort only when we believe that the discomfort will yield some good in the future. If we apply this simple notion to the issue of family care we may ask, "What social and psychological factors pull families toward family care and what factors push them away?" Needless to say, there is a degree of subjectivity in what people value and what they find painful. Each individual and family is unique. Nevertheless, we can offer a few generalizations.

I think it is accurate to say that once the shock of having a developmentally disabled child subsides, most parents show fairly strong motivation to work with and care for their child, at least during the preschool years and the early years of school. With few exceptions, parents just naturally try to care for their offspring, whether handicapped or normal. Society expects this of parents and our socialization process prepares us to expect it of ourselves. We would feel guilty if we didn't try. That doesn't mean that we automatically do a good job or that we assume the parenting role without reluctance or ambivalence. I am simply trying to say that the majority of parents are inclined to care for their handicapped child until such time that they can no longer cope and/or until professionals advise against it. Thus, a primary incentive toward family care is the reality that parents bear a sense of obligation toward the child's well-being. That sense of caring, love, or moral obligation— whatever you chose to call it—may be mixed, of course, with other feelings such as guilt, repulsion, and anger. But my point is that, for most parents, there is a pull toward parenting and family care. If we wish to encourage family care we must recognize that factor, reinforce it and build upon it. In discussing a professional's behavior toward the family, Moyer (1975) makes this same point when she says that:

> Feelings of genuine caring and loving must be identified and allied with in order to achieve family commitment to . . . (early intervention) and developmental growth for the child (p.1).

Most of our public programs and policies do little to recognize and support a family's commitment to care for a handicapped member. Some do the opposite. For example, do we reinforce the concern of middle-income parents when we inform them that their handicapped child is not eligible for Medicaid, Title XX services or SSI so long as he stays home with his family, but that their child would be eligible for these programs if he would leave his family and go into a foster home or a group home?

During the early years of parenting the pull of hope sustains parents because progress, while slow, is fairly tangible (e.g., feeding, crawling, walking, etc.). As the child grows older, progress is less visible and behavior problems become more complex and difficult to handle. Parents begin feeling tired, siblings begin to feel that they are being shortchanged in the family. For parents of normal children, school provides a welcome respite from parenting. For parents of a handicapped child, school is often a hassle. For example, special education programs work hard at involving the parents in programming; as compared to ordinary school programs, a special education program places more demands on the parents. Thus, parents are introduced to social and psychological costs of obtaining services for their child. As compared to the parents of normal children, they must pay a higher price for six hours of relief each school day.

A recurring theme among the frustrations voiced by parents of developmentally disabled children is that the task of being a parent goes on and on. The tasks to be performed by the parent of a handicapped child are both more intensive and extensive. They demand more of the parents for a longer period of time.

When progress is slow and there is little relief from the burdens of parenthood, many parents lose hope. The hopes and joys of parenthood are outweighed by the discomforts and demands. When a crisis occurs they cannot cope. It is at such a time that they request institutionalization or placement into a community-based residential program. Regrettably, the public and many professionals have operated on the basis of what Skarnulis (1976) has termed the "residential assumption," i.e., a person is assumed to need residential services just because he is developmentally disabled. For example, when faced with a family having a difficult time coping with a handicapped member we usually say, in effect, "We realize your burden is great, and getting heavier. Would you like to consider one of our group homes?" In subtle ways this residential assumption has undermined motivation toward family care.

In describing his own experience in designing residential programs, Skarnulis (1976b) stated that:

> . . . A parent seldom came to me saying, "I need my boy out of the house seven days a week." They came to me saying things like, "How can I keep him from scratching his sister?" or "We haven't had a chance to join a bowling league or spend a weekend alone together since Jimmy was born." I begin to wonder if we weren't guilty of overkill. They didn't need residential services, they needed ordinary help just like the rest of us. We went along setting up expensive group homes, institutions and foster homes, then expecting people to fit into them (p. 6).

Let me be quick to point out that Skarnulis is not suggesting that community residential options are unimportant. Rather, he is trying to drive home the point that sometimes our programs undercut the family's motivation for family care. All too often we are forced to offer a family the services we *have* or those that can be funded, but not the ones they really want or *need*.

Because of the way our programs are funded and the type of accountability structure that has evolved, we have become preoccupied with the needs and problems of the handicapped person and tend to forget the rest of the family. For example, the language used in P. L. 94-103 to describe the required habilitation plan creates a rather narrow focus on the training and care of the developmentally disabled individual. I am not opposed to habilitation plans; I am simply pointing out that this language encourages an individual focus, not a family focus. If you look closely at our community programs and services you will find that their focus is on the handicapped member, but not on the needs and the problems of other family members or on the family as a whole. For example, we can provide sophisticated diagnostic services but little in the way of homemaker or chore services. It is quite easy to find funds for a wheelchair but nearly impossible to find money for a washing machine. We can send a handicapped member to camp but cannot help a family have a summer vacation.

During moments of discouragement, when I look at the way we fund family support services and at who is eligible to use them, I wonder if we have created a sort of "psychological means test." You will recall that the way the economic means test works for SSI or Medicaid is that you must spend down or get rid of all your economic resources before you are eligible for financial assistance. Once you have destroyed yourself financially, you become eligible for assistance. It is as if, by placing yourself in genuine financial emergency, you have proven the legitimacy of your claim for outside resources. I see something similar operating in our family support programs. We seem to be able to offer services once the family has nearly destroyed itself or is in a genuine crisis, but don't do much to prevent the destruction in the first place. In a sense, we ask families to "spend down" their emotional and psychological resources before we can offer a relevant service. We ask families to fit our services rather than make our services fit the family.

## CAPACITY

Let's move on to the area I have called capacity. Aside from motivation, what are the prerequisites for successful family care?

A few simple questions will serve to identify some of these and highlight possible incentives and disincentives for family care.

How about time and energy? Family care takes a lot of it. Assuming that support and habilitation services are available, do parents have the time and energy needed to utilize those resources? I think experience demonstrates that if the use of family support services demands more time and energy than it saves, families soon lose interest. It is a simple matter of response cost. The use of support services must make life less hectic, not more hectic.

Do parents and other adults in the household have the capacity to meet the needs of the handicapped member without shortchanging or neglecting the other children in the family?

Do parents, older siblings and others in the household have the knowledge and skills needed to actively participate in individual habilitation plan meetings and carry out their part of the plan?

Do significant family members have whatever it takes to work under professional supervision and learn skills needed to care for a developmentally disabled individual with a severe physical involvement?

Does the family have the financial capacity to handle the extraordinary costs of family care?

Does the family have the ability to cope with neighborhood cranks, public misunderstanding and prejudice against persons who are developmentally disabled?

Do parents and siblings have the energy to fight for the services they need and, when necessary, question the judgments or actions of professionals and agencies?

Are the relationships among all the people in the family, especially the parents' marriage, strong enough to withstand the demands of family care?

Are siblings, especially during the teen years, willing and able to take on some of the family care responsibilities?

Can family members find satisfaction in record keeping, baselining and other activities that are part of home-based service delivery?

Do family members have the objectivity and even the emotional detachment that may be needed to provide a systematic home training and to deal with the behavioral problems of a family member?

Do parents and siblings have the patience and understanding needed to allow their child to experience the joys and anxieties of a sexual awakening during adolescence and early adulthood?

Another way of looking at capacity is to place the question within the context of basic human needs. If we start with the assumption that all people have certain needs and that much of our behavior is an attempt to meet those needs, it follows that unless family members are able to meet their individual needs while being involved in family care, family care is unworkable.

Aside from food, water and shelter, we have a need for physical safety and security; things so basic as decent housing and safety are essential ingredients for family care. We all have a need to be respected and valued. Thus, a family engaged in family care must have the continuing respect and approval of significant others such as friends, relatives, neighbors, employers, etc.; family care must give people a feeling of being worthwhile and useful, but not used. We have a need for affection and for achieving some degree of intimacy with others; family care must not interfere with the development of such relationships. We have a need to know that we are not alone in how we experience life and see the world; family members must be able to discover that others also share in the joys and frustrations of family care, and must not be made to feel that they are alone. Each human being struggles in his own way to figure out what life is all about. There seems to be a need for some kind of a philosophy of life. This may be especially important to persons devoting their life to the care of a handicapped family member. Finally, humans have a need to play, to try out new experiences, to experiment with novelty and do some things just for the hell of it; family care must never become so oppressive or routine that the family loses all spontaneity, humor and sense of adventure. The question for those of us interested in expanding family care becomes one of how we can make it possible for family members to meet those basic human needs, each in his own way, while they assume extraordinary responsibilities.

Additional perspective on the capacity factor becomes apparent when we think about the economically poor family and the so-called multi-problem family. Family care will be particularly difficult for the low income family; the family in poor and overcrowded housing, the family living in an unsafe neighborhood, and the family in which more than one member has serious physical, social or psychological problems. The demands of day-to-day survival for these families are such that there is little time or energy available for the direct care of a seriously handicapped person and the necessary involvement with the many professionals and programs that are a part of habilitative family care.

Systems theory suggests that when a family relationship is unsatisfactory, when the give and take of family life is not meeting the needs of the people in that family, two things commonly happen: (1) the family continues to disintegrate, or (2) the family tries to repair itself through "repeopling." The term "repeopling" is used by some family therapists to describe the family's effort to cope with problems by changing the number of people in the system, by either adding people or excluding people. Asking grandmother to move in with or move out of a family is an example of repeopling. It is a sign that says, "In order to preserve our family system, we must remove one component of the system." What I am trying to suggest is that family care is workable only so long as members of the family can meet their individual needs while engaged in family care. The services used to support family care must somehow tune into those basic human needs and help each family to meet those needs. Stated differently, support services must reduce the negative effect family care may have on an individual's ability to meet his own needs.

Systems theory also tell us that a family attempts to maintain a steady state, a predictable pattern of behavior and activity, that is resistant to change. If that steady state is disrupted, a new one would be established in a matter of weeks or months. This notion of steady state helps to explain why, after a handicapped family member has been placed out of the home, the family usually resists his re-entry into the family system. Once the handicapped member leaves the family, and if there is little or no contact between the individual and the other family members, the family builds a new set of relationships. Each family member establishes a new pattern of need-meeting behavior. Anything that threatens the new family pattern will be resisted. The implication is clear. Once the handicapped family member leaves the family, the possiblity of re-establishing family care is greatly reduced. If we are serious about family care we must be able to provide the supports that prevent initial out-of-home placement. Parenthetically, let me suggest that research in foster care indicates that, once a family member is absent for a year, reintegration becomes increasingly difficult.

## *OPPORTUNITY*

Now a few comments about opportunity. Within the M-C-O Framework, motivation and capacity relate primarily to factors within the family system and between family members. The factor of opportunity applies to what goes on between the individual family and the community. It also applies to forces in wider society, ones well beyond the control of the individual family.

The normalization principle rests on the assumption that, if developmentally disabled individuals live with normal people in normal communities and under normal conditions, they would have more stimulation, more growth experiences, and come as close as possible to achieving their maximum potential. Basically, I agree with that position but, for the purpose of making a point about family behavior, let me say that it "ain't necessarily so."

Butler, Bjaanes and Hofacre (1975) observed that:

> To provide a normalizing environment, community care facilities must provide an environment which is enriched both with internal programs and external contact and exchange. If either is lacking, a deprived environment will tend to develop which will effectively hinder the normalization process (p. 10).

The same thing can be said about family care. Unless the family is enriched by internal programs and by contact and exchange with persons, groups and organizations external to the family, it may offer the handicapped member a deprived environment which provides little stimulation and, in some cases, a highly restricted life experience. Some families, like the old custodial institutions, may encapsulate the developmentally disabled person in an overprotective artificial world. Given the demands of caring for a handicapped person, many families withdraw from contact with others. In order to conserve scarce time and energy, both physical and emotional, the family turns inward and avoids contact with external systems. In doing so, it reduces opportunities for the handicapped person to interact with persons outside the family and the "normal" world beyond the family.

If a family is going to provide habilitative family care, it needs to be involved with professionals, agencies and programs. The dynamics of these relationships must be considered in any serious look at family care. Frequently one hears professionals express frustration and sometimes anger with parents who do not follow the treatment or training plans designed to help the handicapped child. In extreme cases, professionals feel that parents are just getting in the way of sound professional procedures and decisions.

On the other hand, parents often express frustrations and even anger with professionals who make suggestions or design training programs to be carried out by the parent. They say that the plans fail to consider the realities of family life and the heavy demands of maintaining a household. Some parents complain that they are made to feel guilty because they do not do what the professional wants.

In order to "stir up the pot" allow me to offer a few personal observations. Almost by definition, family care means that the parents are the essential and primary providers of care. It is they, not the professionals, who have assumed responsibility for care and training of the handicapped member. Professionals should expect them to behave like parents and family members, not like professionals. Since parents have assumed the responsibility and burden of care, their efforts must be supported and sustained. Professionals must demonstrate trust in and respect for the parents' decisions, their life style, their values and beliefs, and their efforts to care for the handicapped family member. This may mean that professionals have to make some rather significant compromises as to what they think is best for the handicapped individual and what is, for example, good training practice or technique.

We cannot approach family care as if the family was a group home, a special education classroom, or a clinic environment. As Perske (1973) says, there are no ideal families, ". . . there are only messy ones with . . . strengths and weaknesses" (p. 47). Family life is not neat and clean. It is often chaotic with internal conflict.

Family members that provide family care do what they do because they are parents, brothers or sisters and because, in their own unique ways, they care abut the handicapped family member. If a professional treats family members as if they were handmaidens, someone to carry out the professional's order or plan, the professional destroys the very thing he wants to create, i.e., a normal family environment for the handicapped member.

I would like to draw my paper to a close with some remarks about broad societal trends, factors of opportunity far beyond the boundary of the individual family. The American family is undergoing rapid and significant change. There are many types of families. The standard nuclear family (husband, wife and their offspring) is still a dominant form, but only about 37% of the United States families are of that type (Sussman, 1977, p. 359). We must recognize the growing number of single-parent families (one adult plus children), remarried nuclear family (husband, wife and offspring from previous marriages), kin network families (three generation or extended families), and single relative families (composed of single, widowed or divorced relatives living together with children). In addition, there are a growing number of experimental types such as the commune family and unmarried couples with children.

In the process of working on this paper I reviewed some of the mental retardation literature that focused on family dynamics and family support services. With few exceptions, writers discuss parental and sibling reactions, techniques for parent counseling, approaches to home training, etc., as if there were always two parents in the family, as if a handicapped child never acquired stepparents and stepsiblings, and as if the mentally retarded child never experienced the problems of having parents separate or divorce. Needless to say, a divorce or separation has significant short-term and long-term effects on the family's capacity to care for a handicapped member.

Keniston (1977) states that:

> . . . today about one out of every three marriages ends in divorce and more and more of them involve children . . . It is now estimated that four out of every ten children born in the 1970's will spend part of their childhood in a one-parent family, usually with their mother as head of the family (p. 4).

If one includes marriages broken by informal separation and desertion, the rate of family breakup would exceed the one out of three cited above. At least 40% and perhaps 50% of the developmentally disabled children will spend part of their childhood in a one-parent family. Many others will live in families that are different in some way from the traditional nuclear family. Given the demands of caring for a handicapped child, our high rate of family breakup and the growing number of one-parent families may prove to be powerful countervailing forces to any significant expansion of family care.

Inflation and the high cost of living, especially for housing, have pushed a growing number of mothers into the work force. Two incomes have become essential for many families, especially those who want to fulfill the American dream of owning their own home. Families with a developmentally disabled child are not immune from this economic pressure. If anything, they feel it more intensely. In addition to the economic crunch that is pushing mothers into the work force, the women's movement has drawn many mothers out of the home. A growing number of mothers with young children want to move beyond the parent role and find other sources of personal satisfaction. This desire to be something more than just a mother and housewife is also felt by the mothers of developmentally disabled children.

Keniston (1977) states:

> In 1948 . . . only 26 percent of married women with school age children worked at anything but the job of keeping house and raising children. Now that figure has more than doubled: in March 1976 54 percent worked outside the home, a majority of them full time. The increase in labor-force participation is even more dramatic for married women who have preschool age children . . .
>
> . . . we have passed a genuine watershed. This is the first time in our history that the typical school-age child has a mother who works outside the home (p. 4).

These broad social and economic trends are well beyond the influence of national, state or local developmental disabilities programs and planning bodies. They are, however, realities that must be considered. Those who may want to encourage family care must find ways to fund and deliver relevant assistance and support services, regardless of family type or structure. Much of our public policy and many of our public programs are oriented to the nuclear family; non-traditional families have a hard time meeting the eligibility requirements of some programs. We are going to have to be much more innovative and more flexible than in the past and we are going to have to change many state and federal laws and programs that only fit the traditional nuclear family.

## REFERENCES

Sussman, M. Family. In J. Turner, et al., (Eds), *Encyclopedia of Social Work,* Vol. 1. New York: National Association of Social Workers, 1977, 357-368.

Skarnulis, E. Less restrictive alternatives in residential services. *AAESPH Review,* 1976, 1 (3), 40-84.

Moyer, K. Changing family structures for family initiated infant stimulation. Paper presented at the annual meeting of the American Association on Mental Deficiency, Portland, OR, May 1975.

Skarnulis, E. Residential services. Support not supplant the natural home. Paper presented at the Southwestern Region Deaf-Blind Center, Special Study Institute, San Diego, CA, August 22, 1976.

Butler, E., Bjaanes, A., & Hofacre, S. Referral and utilization of services and agencies by community care facilities. Paper presented at the Annual Meeting of the American Association on Mental Deficiency, Portland, OR, May 1975.

Perske, R. *New directions for parents of persons who are retarded.* Nashville: Abingdon Press, 1973.

Keniston, K., & The Carnegie Council on Children. *All our children: The American family under pressure.* New York, Harcourt, Brace, Jovanovich, 1977.

# Sociological Ambivalence and Family Care: The Individual Proposes and Society Disposes

## Bernard Farber

The key question raised by Charles Horejsi in his paper is whether family care is a viable option as a strategy for handling developmentally delayed children. His paper then lays out a series of social and psychological factors "that seem especially relevant to the planning and development of programs designed to support or encourage family care." He organizes these factors in terms of a Motivation-Capacity-Opportunity (M-C-O) framework. Applied to parents of a developmentally disabled child, the framework indicates "that the parents' ability to provide family care is a function of the parents' motivation, their capacity, resources in their immediate environment, and the seriousness and the complexity of the problems presented by the child's handicapping condition." According to the framework, "if you want to maintain the family's ability to provide care while the child's problem becomes more serious, you must provide more and more services in order to increase their motivation, capacity and opportunity."

"Is family care a viable option?" My comments will suggest a response which is different from Horejsi's to this question. I shall first discuss the M-C-O framework as a version of the medical model of treatment applied to social problems. My discussion will imply that, since the model does not focus upon the sources of the social problem, any treatment based on that model is symptomatic and cosmetic. Secondly, my commentary will deal with the prob-

Source: Farber, Bernard. "Sociological Ambivalence and Family Care: The Individal Proposes and Society Disposes." In *Family Care of Developmentally Disabled Members: Conference Proceedings,* edited by Robert H. Bruininks and Gordon G. Krantz. University of Minnesota, 1979. Reprinted with permission.

lem of social contradictions faced by parents of developmentally disabled children. Here, I shall try to show how sociological ambivalences of various kinds impinge upon the destinies of these families and their children. Finally, I shall propose that a more sobering, realistic view may actually enhance the ability of families to cope with their handicapped children. This view takes into account the sociological ambivalences inherent in family relationships.

## *THE M-C-O FRAMEWORK AND THE MEDICAL MODEL*

The medical model of therapy has been enormously successful in the treatment of physical illnesses. According to this model, a practitioner diagnoses an illness or malfunction and prescribes certain medicines or procedures for remediation. Because of these ministrations, the patient is restored to a normal state. Since the model has been so successful in medicine, many social practitioners have applied it to social problems. But its use in the remediation of social dislocations seems to neglect what is truly social and focuses instead upon the "problem persons" themselves. It is mainly this difficulty that I find with the M-C-O framework as a derivative of the medical model.

The phrase "blaming the victim" has become commonplace in social science. The implication, of course, is that the problem at hand is generated by some sort of defect or deficiency in the sufferer himself (or herself). If the deficiency were somehow removed, then the problem would be resolved. This phrase has been applied to a large variety of social problems—racism, sexism, alcoholism, drug abuse, delinquency, and so on. Some people attribute its source to the medical model of treatment; others attribute its derivation to the helping professions in general. Regardless of the source, the personal (or group) deficiency model assumes that a consensus exists as to what is deficient and how to treat it.

The M-C-O framework presented by Horejsi lends itself to the interpretation that it blames the victim—the family of the developmentally disabled child—for its failure to cope with problems of dealing with that child. Not only that, but the family should be encouraged to "normalize" the child and not use him or her in order to solve other difficulties the parents may have. Accordingly, Horejsi proposes that professional services bolster family care whenever family motivations or capabilities are insufficient. However, Horejsi begs the question of criteria of insufficiency.

In indicating the need for preventive measures, Horejsi furthermore suggests that we should not wait for a family to expend itself emotionally—as passing a sort of means test—before providing assistance. Still, a basis must be established for allocating limited resources. Moreover, if respite assistance is to be available to families with retarded chidren, why not others as well—the cerebral palsied, the severely physically handicapped, the invalid parent, the aged? Add to these the possibility that "fraud" is inherent in the medical model. Since there is no consensus on measures for suffering or for "need" for services, we can expect malingerers to make use of the fact that the helping professions are motivated to include questionable cases in the group requiring help. One thus encourages a continual expansion of the helping industry, perhaps geometrically, as "need" expands linearly. Personally, I don't mind this expansion, and in some ways welcome it. But the same kind of overburdening of facilities that occurred for residential institutions may eventually create much dissatisfaction with the helping professions, being so overburdened that their resources are squandered.

The medical model presupposes that motivation and capability reside within people, like gall bladders and livers, and that deficiencies can be compensated for by therapies or respite-help. (See also Lewis, 1978.) The medical perspective ignores the fact that the major factors in adapting to a developmentally delayed child appear to lie outside personal control, in society itself. Larger social forces seem to mold the person's view of how the world operates and of the interpretation of disappointing or noxious events. Motivation and capability are influenced by one's religious beliefs, the parents' educational background, the presence of normal siblings, the existence of supportive kin and friends, and especially interaction in one's own family of orientation (Farber, 1959; 1960; Farber, Jenne, & Toigo, 1960).

In a study dealing with young women's perceptions of what they might do if their children were born grossly deformed, I found that earlier authority patterns in their families of orientation were more effective in predicting their views than were any other concurrent factors, including their life style and present relationships with their parents. The earlier interaction patterns seem to have laid a foundation for their conceptions of legitimate family responsibilities. This earlier family interaction is itself a function of such elements as socioeconomic factors, ethnic and religious background, and other societal variables.

The research sustained the following hypothesized relationships between specific parental authority patterns and daughters' family role orientations:

(a) Egalitarian parental authority in adolescence is associated with the adult daughter's unconditional child orientation, which implies a firm commitment to home care over a career and a rejection of infant euthanasia.

(b) The presence of divided spheres of authority between the teenager's parents is associated with the daughter's later commitment to a strong home role orientation. This orientation gives priority to home care over career, but it does not reject euthanasia of newborns.

(c) Earlier maternal dominance is associated with the grown daughter's "right-to-life" orientation, which gives preference to career over home responsibilities while rejecting euthanasia of newborns.

(d) Paternal dominance is associated with the daughter's unconditional career orientation in adulthood. This orientation not only values career over home responsibilities but also favors euthanasia of grossly deformed newborns.

These findings suggest that the variation in amount of risk that a young woman is willing to take in adapting to a severely defective child is a function of past interaction patterns in her parental home. At one extreme, a young woman from an egalitarian home is more often willing to go all the way in doing whatever is necessary to care for such a child. At the other extreme, the woman whose home had been dominated by her father tends to down-grade home and family responsibility (Farber, 1978).

Even permeability of the family to outside influence is not simply an individual matter related to a motivation to care for the child, family resources, or environmental opportunities. This permeability is influenced in part by religious and ethnic characteristics associated with extended family and communal ties. For instance, Jewish couples, more than others, involve relatives and professionals in their decisions regarding institutionalization of retarded children, Catholics somewhat less, and Protestants least (Farber, Jenne, & Toigo, 1960). This tendency is also revealed in the use of mental health services and concern over children's health (Lurie, 1974; Srole, Langer, Michael, Opler, & Rennie, 1962). The professional role in the decision-making process must obviously vary with the permeability of the family.

To summarize, (1) the M-C-O framework seems to assume that a consensus exists as to what is deficient and how to remedy this deficiency, (2) it would expand the helping industry beyond its capabilities, and (3) it ignores the fact that the major influences in coping with problem children derive from factors which are beyond control of the families.

## SOCIAL CONTRADICTIONS AND PERSONAL PROBLEMS

In dealing with conditions over which families have little control in coping with a severely developmentally disabled child, I propose to focus upon the limitations of assistance intended to alleviate family problems. In doing so, I shall suggest that there are difficulties inherent in long-term family care for the developmentally disabled and that the social context of contemporary society itself operates to counteract attempts at remediation of problems which emerge in the course of family care.

The current world-view with which we operate informs us that, increasingly, technology and modernization of culture have brought a large measure of control over our environment. For a measure of social progress we look to history, and history does reveal many effects of modernization—such as increase in length of life, heightening of quality of life, and greater realization of human potentiality. The decline in infant mortality rates, the virtual elimination of epidemics, and decreases in widespread famine have all lent support to the perspective that we are progressively gaining control over those elements which are destructive to human life and society.

The view that external constraints to the realization of human potential can be dissipated has been extended to personal relationships as well. Contemporary writings on the family emphasize a trend toward the liberation of one's personal life from legal restrictions, moral tradition, and other communal limitations (e.g., Skolnick, 1978). Current ideas about family life are articulated in terms of independence, individual rights, and self-realization. Indeed, this optimistic view has been extended far beyond the reaches of the family into all aspects of contemporary American society. Media of mass communication and mass entertainment promise immediate no-cost gratification, civil rights for all, instant success, a cure for every illness, and an illness for every cure. The notion that all deficiencies can somehow be remedied implies that someone, usually a professional specialist, is available to remove whatever impedes the American Dream. It is my theme that we have oversold the dream.

The plight of families with severely handicapped (especially developmentally delayed) children seems to illustrate the consequences of overselling the American dream. The freedom from constraints about which many writers comment must seem illusory to these families. The parents are caught in a cross-current of contradictions about social expectations. They live in a society which advertises freedom and self-realization on the one hand, but which ascribes tremendous responsibilites for them in caring for their disabled children; they are taught that familial relationships should be fulfilling, and then are presented with a reality which fosters withdrawal and heartache; they are imbued with a concept of childhood that implies development and eventual intellectual maturity, and then are assigned the task of caring for a child who will never attain these aims. The family of the developmentally delayed child is between two worlds, the normal and the deviant, and contradictory social expectations often pull it in opposite directions.

The concept of "sociological ambivalence" can be applied to describe this contradiction. The substance of what Robert K. Merton has called "sociological ambivalence" has endured as a focus of concern over a series of generations. For Merton (1976), "sociological ambivalence in its core sense refers to opposing normative tendencies in the social definition of a role" (p. 12).

In earlier writings, particularly those at the beginning of the twentieth century, sociological ambivalence was seen primarily as an aspect of transition from a feudal society to a modern industrial state. The concept of "the marginal man" was applied by Everett V. Stonequist (1937) not only to "those individuals who fall between two major racial or cultural groups, but also . . . in the relations of minor groups such as social classes, religious sects, and communities." Specifically, the marginal man is one "who through migration, education, marriage, or some other influence leaves one social group or culture without making a satisfactory adjustment to another (and) finds himself on the margin of each but a member of neither" (pp. 2-3). In his depiction of the stranger as a social type, Georg Simmel (1950) observed that the stranger's objectivity in social relations "is a particular structure composed of distance and nearness, indifference and involvement" (p. 404). These opposing tendencies served to give the stranger a unique status and role in a community.

At mid-century, the focus in the study of sociological ambivalence shifted from the transition to an urban society to the complexity of modern social structure. Noting that occupation, income, education, and ethnicity each produce a ranking social status, Gerhard Lenski (1954; 1956) sought to determine the cross-pressures upon individual conduct deriving from inconsistencies in ranking on these attributes. He proposed that "persons with a low degree of status crystallization are more likely to be subjected to disturbing experiences in the interaction process and have greater difficulty in establishing rewarding patterns of social interaction than others" (Lenski, 1956, p. 459). Since then, the consequences of status inconsistencies for mental health, political views, and other attributes have been studied. The contradictions generated by conflicting expectations thus tend to permeate a wide range of relationships. I suspect that these conflicting expectations underlie the persistent profound problems facing families with developmentally delayed children.

Despite the vast increase in services to the developmentally disabled over the past thirty years, the major family problems remain the same. In his paper, Dr. Horejsi remarks, "A recurring theme among the frustrations voiced by parents of developmentally disabled children is that the task of being a parent goes on and on and on." It was this same theme that I heard from parents in the 1950s when I undertook my research on families with severely retarded children and, apparently, it is still prevalent today. In fact, the interpretations of the data that I collected were, in large measure, based upon the proposition that the presence of a severely mentally retarded child in the family inhibits the development of a normal family life cycle. (See also Birenbaum, 1970). My conception of arrest in the family life cycle took the following form:

1. In interaction with their children, parents tend to assign status to each child commensurate with the capabilities they impute to him.
   a. The roles embodied in the status are classified on the basis

of age grading. By definition, normally, mental age is approximately equal to chronological age.

b. Age grading in a culture is regarded more as a psychological and social activity than as a chronological variable, e.g., the chronologically middle-aged severely retarded individual is generally regarded as a "boy" or "girl" by those with whom he interacts.

2. As the child proceeds in his (life) career, the parents normally tend to revise their self-concepts and roles. With respect to their normal children, ideally, parents continually redefine their roles, obligations, and values to adjust to the changing roles of the child. With respect to their retarded children, the parental role is fairly constant. Regardless of his birth order in the family, the severely handicapped child eventually becomes the youngest child socially.

. . . In his progressive movement to the youngest-child status, the severely retarded child would not merely slow down movement in the family cycle but also prevent the development of the later stages in the cycle (Farber, 1968, p. 158, from Farber, 1959).

Drawing upon this conception, I suggested several latent consequences for other family members:

1. A role conflict for siblings, i.e., a partial shifting of roles for the siblings to being caretakers, with a heightened sense of responsibility and possibly resentment for leading a life which suffers by comparison with "childhood" expectations of peers in "normal" families (Farber, 1959; Farber & Jenne, 1963).
2. Being *in* but not part of the "normal" community, i.e., an uneasy sense of difference from other families, especially as the child grows older; often social and occupational withdrawal. Families often maintain their integrity by isolating themselves and giving up the usual criteria for success, such as high sociability or occupational mobility (Culver, 1967; Farber, 1968).
3. The cross-current of home versus career for middle-class women, i.e., keeping the mother in the preschool stage maternal role, the period of motherhood in which outside occupations are least sought. Hence, mothers would be less likely to seek outside employment.

4. Concern of future contradictions, i.e, depending upon the parents' orientation toward the future, some parents would anticipate the arrest of the family cycle rather than merely experience it. While they all would try to develop strategies for counteracting its effects, for many the enormity of the domestic tragedy which the future held would lead to much mental anguish. Since middle-class parents more often than working-class parents focus upon the future, one would expect this anguish of anticipated family-cycle arrest to occur mainly in middle-class families (Farber, 1960.)

In his discussion of structural sociological ambivalence, Merton directs our attention to the conflicting demands inherent in a single role. These demands, he writes, generate oscillation between conflicting aspects of a social relationship. For example, every non-ascriptive (i.e., revocable) social relationship must at the same time establish norms for fulfilling whatever tasks are involved, and simultaneously it must also contain the seeds for its own destruction—how is the relationship to be brought to a conclusion legitimately? Children vacillate in-between parents and peers seeking approval over their actions; lovers manufacture quarrels; subordinates test the limits of tolerance. In revocable relationships, there must be a point at which the destructive elements are supposed to predominate. Merton (1976) suggests that "this alternation of subroles *evolves* as a social device for helping people in designated statuses to cope with the contingencies they face in trying to fulfill their functions" (p. 18). An undercurrent of conflict and quarreling is more threatening to a life-long relationship than in a voluntary, fleeting one not only because of the discomfort it may produce but also because this undercurrent signals to the participants the fact that, in a significant way, the relationship resembles a revocable one.

The conception of arrest in the family life-cycle may also reveal something about the long range consequences of the presence of a developmentally disabled child in the home. For the severely developmentally disabled person, norms in the family of orientation do not provide an opportunity for revocation. Hence, the ordinary signals for revocability may become a threat to the strength of the bonds between the disabled person and his (or her) parents and siblings; instead of welcoming even a limited development of social and economic independence, emergence of quarrels and conflict, and growing apart emotionally, parents may want to suppress them in order to make life a little easier over the years. It is little wonder that parents of developmentally disabled children are frequently seen by educators, psychologists, and social workers as overly protective.

Perhaps the most significant consequence of the absence of the norm of revocability of domestic roles is the frustration of normalization of the disabled child. The lack of an undercurrent of revocability in turn leads to problematic terminations of familial ties. In the book, *Cloak of Competence*, Robert Edgerton (1967) sets forth the proposition that adult mentally retarded persons generally are able to live in community settings because of the continual sponsorship of a parental surrogate—a relative, a close friend, a neighbor, an employer, a social worker, and so on. This person acts as a manager of the retarded person's personal, employment, and financial affairs. But Cunningham (1976) suggests that:

> Sponsorship, however, seems to be a two-edged sword: it provides a series of benefits to the person sponsored, but it may also limit the potential adult role performance of the person sponsored and . . . may be withdrawn by the sponsor at the sponsor's option. As with most roles which include dependence on another, the retarded person live(s) a precarious existence (p. 65).

Hence, without an undercurrent of norms signalling the legitimacy of revocability of domestic roles in the case of developmentally disabled children, several problems emerge: (1) role contradictions stemming from arrest in the family cycle, (2) the overprotectiveness by the parents, (3) uncertainties in the later stages of the family life-cycle, and (4) the handicapped person's being at the mercy of the parental surrogate's good will. The social contradictions which impinge upon families with severely mentally handicapped children seem to amplify the ambivalences and cross-currents which other families ordinarily endure.

## BRINGING SOCIAL REALITY BACK IN: THE NORMALITY OF DISAPPOINTMENT

In the past thirty years, how much have we done to assist parents of developmentally disabled children? No matter how we disguise a bitter pill, it is still a bitter pill. We can use linguistic subterfuges; we can offer sops of "respite care" in order to co-opt parents;

we can give special training to parents and siblings to help cope with everyday contingencies; we can organize parents to commiserate with each other over their disabled children and to seek common solutions for an unending list of problems. We can do all these, but we cannot eliminate the idea of tragedy and disappointment. Dr. Horejsi tells us that, when all is said and done, the responsibility for the developmentally disabled child rests with the parents, that "the very thing we are trying to achieve . . . (is) allowing the handicapped person to live with his or her family." With the closing off of institutional admissions, parents are more often forced into family care; the child is there, and all we can do for the parents, as in the case of the terminal cancer patient, is to make life a little more palatable and to ease the pain. But at the same time, we subtly inform the parents that if they cannot cope with the problems of handling their developmentally delayed children, they themselves are somehow defective or deficient.

Because of modern technological advances, we all are led to exaggerated expectations in every area of existence. During the last part of the nineteenth century, the rapid economic development in Western society gave rise to the myths of open upward economic and social mobility. Today, a similar optimism seems to pervade the society in areas of personal relationships. Many observers attribute the current high divorce rate and the continual seeking of alternative domestic life styles to the exaggeration of expectations of what one should get out of marriage and family life. Indeed, one of the consequences of isolation of family units is the ignorance of the frustrations and disappointments that go on in other families. Privacy in the contemporary family not only permits "alternative life styles," but is also enables people to display an "optimistic" and "happy" front to the world. Most important, this "optimism" of exaggerated expectations becomes the norm, the model of domestic existence. This is the social context in which the parents of a severely disabled child find themselves. People are led to believe that suffering is abnormal, that any disappointment constitutes some sort of deviance.

Still, whereas technological control has advanced with incredible speed, most of us can expect to endure much disappointment and suffering during our lifetimes. Despite our emphasis upon the achievement of "success"—family success, educational success, economic success, and, mainly, success in interpersonal relations—there is no earthly paradise, there is no "soma" pill, and no solution for many problems. All relationships—even between the helping professionals and their clients—have elements of disappointment. One might say that disappointment is a necessary undercurrent, a negative aspect of a sociological ambivalence, in any sustained interaction. Some of us are luckier than others and have an obligation to diffuse our luck. But we also have an obligation not to try to oversell our product, our assistance to the unlucky.

Without acceptance of disappointment as "normal," as Emile Durkheim recognized almost a century ago, human wants are insatiable and, as a consequence, when dreams are not realized, despair is deepened. The normality of disappointment seems to have disappeared in the optimism of the twentieth century; with its disappearance, the burdens of failure are magnified. It is not merely motivation and resources, but also what the family *expects* to happen that determines the kind of environment it can provide in caring for the developmentally disabled child. Parents are led to maintain their illusion that a worldly Nirvana or secular grace is possible. Failure to recognize the inherent contradictions in all social relations serves to heighten problems in families with developmentally disabled children. In refusing to consider disappointment and tragedy as normal modes of existence (as concomitants of achievement), we magnify frustration and suffering for families with disabled children: We then blame them for failing to achieve the Modern Dream.

## REFERENCES

Lewis, M. *The culture of inequality.*Amherst: The University of Massachusetts Press, 1978.
Farber, B. Effects of a severely mentally retarded child on family integration. *Monographs of the Society for Research in Child Development,* 1959, 24, No.2.
————. Perceptions of crisis and related variables in the impact of a retarded child on the mother. *Journal of Health and Social Behavior,* 1960, 1, 108-118.
————, Jenne, W.C., & Toigo, R. Family crisis and the decision to institutionalize the retarded child. *Council for Exceptional Children Monograph Series.* Series A, Number 1, 1960.
————. Parental decision-making: Justifying transgressions. In C.A. Swinyard (Ed.), *Decision-making and the defective newborn.* Springfield: Charles C. Thomas, 1978, 123-157.
Lurie, O.R. Parents' attitudes toward use of mental health services. *American Journal of Orthopsychiatry,* 1974, 44, 109-120
Srole, L., Langer, T.S., Michael, S.T., Opler, M.K., & Rennie, T.A. *Mental health in the metropolis.* New York: McGraw-Hill, 1962.
Skolnick, A. *The intimate environment: Exploring marriage and the family.* Boston: Little, Brown, 1978.
Merton, R.K. *Sociological ambivalence and other essays.* New York: Free Press, 1976.

Stonequist, E.V. *The marginal man.* New York: Charles Scribner's Sons, 1937.

Simmel, G. *The sociology of Georg Simmel.* New York: Free Press, 1950.

Lenski, G.E. Status crystallization: A non-vertical dimension of social status. *American Sociological Review,* 1954, 19, 405-413.

———. Social participation and status crystallization. *American Sociological Review,* 1956, 21, 458-464.

Birenbaum, A. On managing courtesy stigma. *Journal of Health and Social Behavior,* 1970, 11, 196-206.

Farber, B. *Mental retardation: Its social context and social consequences.* Boston: Houghton Mifflin, 1968.

——— and Jenne, W.C. Interaction with retarded siblings and life goals of children. *Journal of Marriage and the Family,* 1963, 25, 96-98.

Culver, M. Intergenerational social mobility among families with a severely mentally retarded child. Unpublished Ph.D. dissertation, University of Illinois, Urbana, 1967.

Farber, B. Perceptions of crisis and related variables in the impact of a retarded child on the mother. *Journal of Health and Social Behavior,* 1960, 1, 108-118.

Merton, R.K. *Sociological ambivalence and other essays.* New York: Free Press, 1976.

Edgerton, R.B. *The cloak of competence.* Berkeley: University of California Press, 1967.

Cunningham, J.J. Institutionalization of post-school aged retarded persons of mild and borderline intelligence. Unpublished Ed.D. dissertation, University of Illinois, Urbana, 1975.

# Community Care and Deinstitutionalization: A Review

Steven P. Segal

The policy of returning mental patients to their own communities assumes that the family will support individuals who can barely take care of their personal needs. However, few attempts have been made to specify the joint functions of the mental hospital and the family in providing care in the community for the mentally ill. Furthermore, little effort has been made to cite the responsiblities delegated to the family in the context of community care. Finally, there have been few attempts to elaborate on the social policies of community care and deinstitutionalization. This article addresses these issues, reviews the research related to the family as a helper in community care, and makes suggestions as to what the policies should be with respect to the family's role in this vital area.

## GOALS AND FUNCTIONS

The concept of community care is an old one. It was reintroduced in the early 1930s as an adjunct of state hospital care. One of the goals of community care is to shift the responsibility for the care of patients from the institution to the community, with the institution acting in a supportive role to local mental health and social agencies, recreation and police departments, and the like. These community agencies coordinate their efforts to support the family in providing the care needed by the released patient. During the late 1950s and early 1960s, innovative state hospital programs such as that implemented by the Dutchess County Unit of Hudson River State Hospital in Poughkeepsie, New York, maintained as many as two-thirds of their inpatients in the community. This unit instituted an easy-in and easy-out policy through which the hospital supported but not necessarily housed the patients. Its major goal was to help patients maintain their social role in the family.

Another goal of community care is to prevent chronic disabilities that are attributable to prolonged periods in locked wards of under-staffed and poorly run mental institutions. In the 1960s and early 1970s, however, this goal became confused with the policy of deinstitutionalization, which involves the removal of the mentally ill from mental instututitions. Although the goals of deinstitutional-ization are to prevent chronic disability, protect patients' rights, and reduce the cost of care, hospitalized mental patients have been moved to communities without the provision of supportive net-works in the community. For many of these released patients the cost of leaving the mental hospital has not been as great as the negative impact of the institution itself; for others costs have been considerable. The latter individuals have often been placed in com-munities in which they are unwanted and consequently become more isolated from social relationships than they had been in the hospital.

Gruenberg (1970) outlines the following functions of the mental hospital in providing short-term treatment of the mentally ill: (1) to use treatment procedures that require continuous observation, (2) to protect patients who endanger themselves or others, (3) to remove persons temporarily from an environmental stress during a period when they cannot cope with the stress, (4) to provide temporary relief for those who manage to live with patients, and (5) to estab-lish communication between patients and the hospital.

In addition to these functions, the mental hospital has served as a primary provider of long-term mental health care to the aged, as maintainer of the physical and mental health of the chronically mentally ill, and as a supportive social community (often with many negative factors associated with it) for the chronic population. These responsibilities, however, have been shifted back to the family, leaving primarily those functions outlined by Gruenberg (1970) to the mental hospital.

In considering the responsibilities delegated to the family in the care of the mentally ill, these questions must be raised: What is the readiness of the family to accept these responsibilities? What is the impact of these responsibilities on the ongoing relationships in the family and on the long-term adjustment of the patients to the community? In view of these questions, the supportive role of the family can be examined in terms of three levels of prevention: primary, secondary, and tertiary. The author discusses each level, starting with the third.

## TERTIARY PREVENTION

Tertiary prevention includes community and family planning that leads to prevention of long-term chronic disability and "institutionalism," that is, dependence on and total orientation toward the mental institution. Research has shown that it is possible to achieve these two goals (Segal, 1978). However, is the family ready, able, and willing to provide support for the chronic mental patient? To answer this question, the author will consider the following: (1) the current availability of family support for chronic mental patients, (2) the willingness of the family to assume the additional responsibility for the patient, (3) the impact of assuming these responsibilities on the family, and (4) the relationship between the placement of patients in a family context in the community and the prevention of chronic disability and institutionalism.

### Availability of Family Support

Although only a small proportion of all admissions to mental hosptials in any given cohort of admissions is isolated or has little support available to it, this proportion becomes the large residual population of chronic mental patients in the mental health system. Each progressive cohort of returns to a mental hospital has a larger percentage of people in the cohort who have no family support or who have a limited amount of interaction with family members. (Miller, 1965; Pasamanick, Scarpitti, and Dinitz, 1967; and Davis, Dinitz, and Pasamanick, 1974).

In a study of former mental patients, aged 18-65, living in community-based sheltered-care facilities in California, Segal and Aviram (1978) found that 52 percent of the patients rarely, if ever, had access to family members. In addition, 60 percent had never been married, 35 percent had dissolved their relationships, and only 5 percent were married. When examined by sex, these figures revealed that 73 percent of the men as opposed to 44 percent of the women had never been married, 22 percent of the men and 50 percent of the women were either separated or divorced, and only 4 and 5 percent of the men and women, respectively, were married.

These figures reflect a pattern that is characteristic of the population who require long-term institutional care. As any given cohort becomes increasingly involved with the mental health system, its marital status begins to approximate those described previously. Given these statistics, the question must be raised as to the extent to which the family is available to meet the needs of the truly chronic patient.

### *Willingness of the Family to Assume Additional Responsibility*

To some extent the attitude of family members toward the ex-patient reflects their willingness to assume responsibility for a relative returning after a prolonged hospitalization or several short hospitalizations. Previous studies have shown that the attitudes of family members toward released patients seem to be significantly more positive and accepting than those expressed by members of society as a whole (Philips, 1963; Schwartz, Myers, and Astrachan, 1974; and Swanson and Spitzer, 1970).

Another indicator of a family's desire to assume such responsibility is its expressed willingness to accept the discharged relative back in the home. Research on this subject addresses three aspects. The first aspect relates to the family's attitude toward the return of the patient from the hosptial; the second, to the family's attitude toward the former patient after he or she has been living in the home awhile; and the third, to the psychological, financial, economic, and social burdens placed on the family by accepting the relative back in the home.

When looking at the first aspect, Rose (1959) observed an increasing reluctance on the part of families to accept discharged patients in the home as the number of years of hospitalization increased. In addition, Evans, Bullard, and Solomon (1961) reported that less than 50 percent of the families they interviewed favored the release of their relatives who had been hospitalized for five years or more. On the other hand, Freeman and Simmons (1963) reported that 95 percent of their family members wanted the patients to live in their household. And Wing and his associates (1964) found that no family members refused to take back their discharged relatives, although 13 percent actively opposed their return and 21 percent were doubtful about it.

Three related factors influence the family's willingness to accept the former patient: the severity of the patient's symptoms, pessimism about the ability of the patient to recover, and stressful conditions in the environment that are related to lower social-class status. Findings reported by Doll (1976) revealed a relationship between the rate of rejection of discharged patients by family members and the onset of severe symptoms. For example, although 83 percent of all the familes studied said they wanted the discharged patients to come home, 58 percent of those with severely disturbed relatives opposed their return. In addition, 71 percent who wanted to exclude discharged patients from their social lives were living with severely disturbed former patients. Moreover, Swingle (1965) indicated that half the families of a group of mental patients believed that the patients could not recover from their illness and thus were unable to return home. In addition, Hollingshead and Redlich (1958) found that members of the lowest social class were most unwilling to accept their discharged relatives in the home.

When faced with the actual responsibility of having a discharged relative in the home, however, families seem to respond better to the patient. Barrett, Kuriansky, and Gurland (1972) found that of 85 families whose relatives had returned home following a hospital strike in New York State, 60 percent expressed pleasure about their return. In addition, Brown and his associates (1966), in their study of 251 families, found that five years after the relatives' discharge, 75 percent of the families welcomed the patients in the household, 15 percent accepted them and only 12 percent wanted them to live elsewhere.

## Cost to the Family for Being a Caretaker

The key issue as reported in several studies on this subject is the extent to which the former patient actually places a burden on the family. For example, Grad and Sainsbury (1963a, 1963b, and 1968) noted that 81 percent of the families who rejected their discharged relatives had economic and social problems, whereas only 62 percent of those who accepted the former patients had such problems. Moreover, Barrett, Kuriansky, and Gurland (1972) reported that when patients placed no burden on the household, they were more likely to remain in the home and thus stay out of the hospital. However, in his study, Doll (1976) found that 67 percent of the family members interviewed were ashamed because they had a severely disturbed relative living at home.

In view of the cost to the family for housing a former patient, family members seem to tolerate a great deal of disruption. Hoenig and Hamilton (1969) reported on 179 families who lived continuously with a former patient for four years prior to the research interview. These researchers compared the "subjective" reports of burden made by families with the "objective" rating of burden made by a social worker. They concluded that there was a great deal of subjective tolerance in view of the objective rating of a heavy burden experienced by families. Although 90 percent of the families in the study were sympathetic toward the patient, 56 percent of them expressed relief when the relative was admitted to the mental hospital.

## *Prevention of Chronic Social Disability and Institutionalism*

Research shows that the family plays a role in preventing as well as contributing to the development of long-term chronic social disability and institutionalism. For example, a study by Barrett, Kuriansky, and Gurland (1972) demonstrated a significant relationship between the attitude of family members toward discharged patients and the amount of time patients remained in the community. Results showed that 57 percent of the relatives of the patients who did not require rehospitalization were initially pleased with the patient's release and only 7 percent of the relatives of those who were rehospitalized responded in this way.

In addition, a study by Greenley (1979) showed that discharged patients were more likely to be rehospitalized if their families expected them to have few friends outside the family, to create a childlike situation in the home, or to exhibit severe psychiatric symptoms. Greenley hypothesized that two types of dependent relationships existed between ex-patients and their families: the ambivalent and inconsistent and the ineffective and rejecting types, both of which involve a basic dislike and rejection of the patient. This hypothesis is consistent with the clinical observations of Stein and his associates (1975) who reported that repeated hospitalizations were a result of a pathological relationship between the patient and family. To deter such a relationship and prevent rehospitalization, these researchers are in favor of separating the patient from the family.

Other researchers also revealed that a relationship exists between the family's interactions with former patients and the readmission rate. For example, Brown and his colleagues (1958, 1962, and 1972) explored the emotional arousal hypothesis. This hypothesis suggests that some environments, which include the mother or wife, are too emotionally stimulating for ex-patients. Therefore, former patients living with their mothers or wives may have a higher readmission rate than those living with siblings, with distant kin, or in lodgings. Findings not only supported the hypothesis but also indicated that there was an optimal level of emotional arousal above which patients were more likely to return to the hospital.

Early studies by Freeman and Simmons (1958 and 1959) generated the tolerance-of-deviance hypothesis. This hypothesis assumes that families with a high tolerance will continue to accept former patients even when they fail to perform tasks related to work and housekeeping. These researchers found that fewer relapses occur among patients living with families that have low expectations regarding patients' performance. But later studies by Freeman and Simmons (1963), Angrist and her colleagues (1968), and Michaux and his associates (1969) failed to demonstrate a relationship between tolerance of deviance and the amount of time a patient spent in the community.

However, the results of a study by Greenley (1979) supported a hypothesis concerning families' tolerance of symptoms. It was found that former patients who were rehospitalized at a faster rate than others lived with families that had a low tolerance for the expression of symptoms. Although further research is needed to replicate the findings of these various studies, there is reason to believe that a properly selected family environment can contribute to the length of time a patient spends in the community and thus to the prevention of long-term chronic social disability.

Factors that may contribute to the development of institutionalism are social isolation and the limited housing options available to a person. Institutionalism is not necessarily confined to the mental institution. Segal and Moyles (in press) reported that a significant proportion of the mentally ill residents in community care facilities developed a dependence on these facilities. In addition, Brown and his associates (1962) observed that discharged chronic patients who lived with their families were totally isolated in the home and evidenced behaviors associated with institutionalism. Thus, internal aspects of the family as well as the institutional environment are crucial in preventing the development of institutionalism among ex-patients.

## SECONDARY PREVENTION

Secondary prevention seeks to reduce the negative effects of mental illness by early diagnosis and treatment. The family can help patients by maintaining its role structure, thereby short-circuiting any attempts to exclude and thus deprive patients of performing normal family roles. As discussed previously, prolonged hospitalization is related to the increasing reluctance of a family to accept the patient in the home. In addition, researchers have offered other explanations for the reluctance of family members to accept patients. Pitt (1960), for example, argued that former patients exhaust a "reservoir of good will" toward themselves. And Dunigan (1969) concluded that there is a critical point at which the family's expectations of the patient's performance and the family's tolerance of deviant behavior change. Men coped well with one or two hospitalizations of their wife or mother. But with more than three hospitalizations, they tended to withdraw from their female relative, lower their expectations, and make more permanent changes in their household to allow for continued functioning without the presence of the female (Kreisman and Joy, 1974).

Mills (1962) pointed out that when the stress of having a mentally ill relative in the home became too great, families turned to the hospital for relief. Rehospitalization was often followed by a deterioration of the relationship between the patient and his or her family. Myers and Bean (1968) found similar results in their follow-up study, noting that the deterioration of relationships following rehospitalization was true in lower-class families.

Visiting is a crucial element to consider when examining the involvement of the family with hospitalized patients. Rawnsley, Loudon, and Miles (1962) studied records of 230 private patients. They found that 20 percent of the patients had no contact with their families outside the hospital. In addition, the key factor in determining rates of visitation was the length of time patients spent in the hospital. The longer the patient spent in the hospital, the less they were visited. Sommer (1958 and 1959) also found that those patients who were hospitalized longer had fewer visitors and less correspondence with their family. Furthermore, Myers and his associates (1959 and 1968) reported less visiting and gift-giving among lower-class families.

It is unclear whether the family members' failure to visit and their rejection of the mental patient are synonymous. In some studies they are (Alivisatos and Lykestos, 1964; and Myers and Bean, 1968). In others they seem to be independent (Gillas and Keet, 1965; and Rose, 1959). However, visiting and the family's involvement with the patient are related to negotiating the patient's release from the mental hosptial, for it is the family who often negotiates the discharge.

An indicator of the restructuring of the family to exclude the ex-mental patient is the divorce rate of former mental patients. Adler (1955) found that divorce and separation rates among mental patients were three times higher than the national average. In addition, in a study of Puerto Rican couples, Rogler and Hollingshead (1965) noted that fewer spouses of schizophrenics said that they would remarry the same person to which they were currently married than did spouses of "normals".

These findings suggest that patients will have problems when trying to maintain their position in society and in the family. Thus, the absence of patients over time is crucial in determining their slow exclusion from the ongoing family process in which they were previously involved.

## *PRIMARY PREVENTION*

From the perspective of primary prevention, the family is delegated two roles: that of helping to define illness and that of providing the social supports necessary to protect individuals from stressful conditions in the environment that can contribute to the development of mental disorders. Often the family is reluctant to define the relative's problem as mental illness and consequently does not make the initial diagnosis. The crucial element here in relation to the family's functioning is the attempt of the family to explain the relative's behavior in a normal frame of reference. It is unclear, however, what the consequences of the normalization process are. Although this process may delay treatment for many serious cases, it may also serve as a supportive device for milder cases and as a preventive measure in the labeling of patients. Therefore, much more research is needed on the role of the family in the normalization and diagnostic processes.

"Social margin" refers to the set of skills, resources, and relationships one draws on to survive in society. It is one's "social bank account" that enables him or her to cope with stress. The family is one's major and enduring source of social margin. It is the source of one's biological inheritance, interactional skills, and significant others who function as a support system to help

> . . . the individual mobilize his psychological resources and master his emotional burdens, share his tasks, and provide him with extra supplies of money, materials, tools, skills, and cognitive guidance . . . (Caplan, 1974, p. 6).

Loss of a family member through death or divorce, genetic predisposition, and intrafamilial patterns of interaction have all been implicated as factors affecting one's risk of developing a pyschological disorder.

More specifically, with respect to the role of the family in providing social support, the longitudinal study of Kellum, Ensminger, and Turner (1977) is most important. These researchers delineated as many as sixty-eight family structures on the basis of different combinations of household members who lived in an urban area in Chicago. They pointed out that these different combinations were able to provide different levels of support for their children and therefore were differentially able to insulate them from the environmental stresses related to mental disorders. Furthermore, they noted that children in single-parent families faced greater threats to their psychological well-being than did those in other familial structures. The former encountered more threats because of the limited availability of social supports. However, in families in which the presence of a second relative served as an enabling or protective resource similar to that of the traditional nuclear family, the risks for mental illness were significantly reduced.

In addition, Robins found that

> children raised by both their own parents were more often well than other children, and children for whom responsibility was vested outside the parents were least often well (1966, p. 174).

Although this finding was attributed solely to the virtual nonexistence of an antisocial father in cases in which children were reared by both parents, it raises questions about the importance of support systems in the maintenance of psychological well-being. However, little is known about the role of the family as a support system in helping individuals to cope with the precipitators of mental disorders.

# IMPLICATIONS

## Policies That Support Tertiary Prevention

The original study of Pasamanick, Scarpitti, and Dinitz (1967) demonstrated that mental hospitalization could be prevented by administering antipsychotic medications to discharged patients. However, it was conducted with individuals who had intact families, not with long-term chronic patients who were often without family support. This suggests the need for the development of substitute family units, along with accompanying service supports, as an alternative for long-term chronic patients. Such substitute environments as small group homes and long-term care facilities that do not resemble institutions but are more family oriented should be organized and funded. To accomplish this, Section 8 of HUD (Housing and Urban Development) Subsidized Housing Programs could be expanded.

In addition, a true system of community care is needed rather than one that simply emphasizes the moving of people out of institutions into the community without proper social supports. The planning of activities for discharged patients should be an essential element in the system. Such planning could be conducted in coordination with a mental hospital or with a local community mental health center.

An implication of research on community care relates to the amount of burden absorbed by families who take on the responsibility of their chronically mentally ill relatives. For these families, options related to respite care must be considered. In the past, as previously noted, the hospital served as a temporary relief for patients who could not cope successfully with stressful conditions in their environment and for family members who lived with patients at significant cost to themselves. Either the hospital could again be used in this way, emphasizing an easy admission and easy discharge policy, or "crisis houses" in the community could be set up to fulfill this function. Crisis houses would probably be more desirable because of their location in the community and the nonmedical label attached to such facilities. The latter might be most helpful in preventing the occurrence of any iatrogenic effects associated with being in the hospital.

Another implication related to the reduction of burden on the family suggests the need for the development of a sound supportive social work program. Grad and Sainsbury (1963a, 1963b, and

1968) compared a traditional hospital program with a community care program. They observed that relatives of patients in the community care program experienced many more burdens than relatives of patients in the traditional hospital program. In addition, the major factor that influenced the amount of burden experienced by the family was the regular visits made to the home by the social work staff of the traditional program. It thus seems that a community care program that provides supportive social work services can be effective in reducing the amount of burden placed on the family.

In considering institutionalization, the problem of sheltered-care facilities or family households as community back wards should be addressed. To cope with this situation, policies are needed that aim at creating educational programs for community care workers and relatives of chronic mental patients. These programs should emphasize that social isolation in sheltered-care facilities or the family could lead to the development of the same type of dependencies experienced in the mental institution and could have negative effects on family life. They should further emphasize that the high expectations of workers and family members would enable former patients to fulfill their maximum potential.

In view of the emotional involvement of patients with other family members, someone should determine whether patients would function better in a sheltered-care facility than in the family unit. A social worker could make this determination and help the family work through its own needs and involvements with the former patient. This suggests, therefore, the need for a strong locally based unit of social workers who would develop optimal placements and provide supportive services to chronic mental patients living in the home or in community care facilities.

## Policies That Support Secondary Prevention

To prevent the exclusion of former patients from the family, the hospital and other supportive facilities such as crisis houses should function as short-term resources in providing community care. Patients who return to these facilities for brief periods of time should not be viewed as failures but as persons who want to cope with their illness in an institutional setting. Without doubt the easy-in and easy-out policy being advocated here places a burden on the family, especially in the area of work and social activities. Therefore, the family should receive supportive community services during the inital stressful periods of brief hospitalization.

Unfortunately, some patients may be unable to resume their previous level of work and social-role functioning. In this case, supports should be offered to other family members in meeting the demands of some of the roles previously performed by the patient. For example, work training programs could be offered to the wives of released patients who have experienced repeated hospitalizations and who seem to be suffering from a more or less permanent or total disability. This type of program might help the family maintain its commitment to the former patient and reduce the amount of pessimism and disillusionment often associated with helping the long-term chronic patient. Although a change in roles can create a significant amount of stress for individuals in the family, people often rise above stressful situations and maximize the potential of these situations for their own growth.

In addition, as part of the general orientation toward community care, social workers should help family members understand the fine line between maintaining realistic expectations and maintaining a "high expectation environment." The former prevents the disillusionment of family members; the latter prevents patients from drifting into chronic dependence and enables them to fulfill their potential. Although these may seem to be contradictory goals, the "fine tuning" of the balance betweem them is crucial to enhanced patient outcome.

### Policies That Support Primary Prevention

Further research should examine the role of the family as a diagnoser of mental illness, especially the family's attempt to normalize all behavior before recognizing the presence of illness. In addition, education programs that promote a positive understanding of mental disorder should continue to be sponsored by federal agencies. These programs should include materials that illustrate the importance of the family in supporting the mentally ill. Finally, the social supports necessary to prevent the development of psychological problems should be provided. These supports should include child care and programs that enable single parents to exchange supportive activities and perhaps serve as an extended family.

After one hundred years the family is once again being asked to assume its major function as care-giver for the long-term mentally ill patient. If it is to assume this role meaningfully, the community care movement must take the word *care* seriously. The community must provide professional manpower, professional expertise, and social activities. If such supports do not become available, the mentally ill will be rejected by the general community and their families and will live primarily isolated existences in isolated settings. Their lives will perhaps not be too far removed from the lives of other mental patients who were found in the back wards of large mental hospitals or who were rescued from the jails by Dorothea Dix.

## BIBLIOGRAPHY

*Readers will note that bibliographical style has been used for references in this article. It is used only for reviews of the literature.*

Adler, Leta M. "Patients of a State Mental Hospital: The Outcome of their Hospitalization," in Arnold M. Rose, ed., *Mental Health and Mental Disorder*. New York: W. W. Norton & Co., 1955. Pp. 501-523.

Alivisatos, Gerassimos, and Lykestos, George. "A Preliminary Report of a Research Concerning the Attitude of the Families of Hospitalized Mental Patients," *International Journal of Social Psychiatry,* 10 (Winter 1964), pp. 37-44.

Angrist, Shirley, et al. *Women After Treatment.* New York: Appleton-Century-Crofts, 1968.

Barrett, James E.; Kuriansky, Judith; and Gurland, Barry. "Community Tenure Following Emergency Discharge," *American Journal of Psychiatry,* 128 (February 1972), pp. 958-964.

Brown, George; Birley, J. L. T.; and Wing, John. "Influence of Family Life in the Course of Schizophrenic Disorders: A Replication," *British Journal of Psychiatry,* 121 (September 1972), pp. 241-258.

Brown, George; Carstairs, G.M.; and Topping, Gillian. "Post Hospital Adjustment of Chronic Mental Patients," *Lancet,* 7048, No. 2 (September 27, 1958), pp. 685-689.

Brown, George, et al. "Influence of Family Life on the Course of Schizophrenic Illness," *British Journal of Prevention and Social Medicine,* 16 (April 1962).

Brown, George, et al. *Schizophrenia and Social Care.* New York: Oxford University Press, 1966.

Caplan, Gerald. *Support Systems and Community Mental Health.* New York: Behavioral Publications, 1974. P. 6.

Davis, Ann; Dinitz, Simon; and Pasamanick, Benjamin. *Schizophrenics in the Custodial Community: Five Years After the Experiment.* Columbus, Ohio: Ohio State University Press, 1974.

Doll, William. "Family Coping with the Mentally Ill: An Unanticipated Problem of Deinstitutionalization," *Hospital and Community Psychiatry,* 27 (March 1976), pp. 183-185.

Dunigan J. "Mental Hospital Career and Family Expectations." Unpublished manuscript, Laboratory of Psychosocial Research, Cleveland Psychiatric Institute, 1969.

Evans, Anne S.; Bullard, Dexter M.; and Solomon, Maida H. "The Family as a Potential Resource in the Rehabilitation of the Chronic Schizophrenic Patient," *American Journal of Psychiatry,* 117 (June 1961), pp. 1075-1083.

Freeman, Howard, and Simmons, Ozzie. "Mental Patients in the Community: Family Settings and Performance Levels," *American Sociological Review,* 23 (April 1958), pp. 147-154.

————. "Social Class and Posthospital Performance Levels," *American Sociological Review,* 24 (June 1959), pp. 345-351.

————. *The Mental Patient Comes Home.* New York: John Wiley & Sons, 1963.

Gillas, L. S., and Keet, M. "Factors Underlying the Retention in the Community of Chronic Rehospitalized Schizophrenics." *British Journal of Psychiatry,* 11 (November 1965), pp. 1057-1067.

Grad, Jacqueline, and Sainsbury, Peter. "Evaluating a Community Care Service," in Hugh L. Freeman and James Farndale, eds., *Trends in Mental Health Service.* Elmsford, N.Y.: Pergamon Press, 1963a. Pp. 303-317.

————. "Mental Illness and the Family," *Lancet,* 7280, No. 1 (March 9, 1963b), pp. 544-547.

————. "Effects that Patients Have on their Families in a Community Care and a Control Psychiatric Service—A Two Year Following," *British Journal of Psychiatry,* 114 (March 1968), pp. 265-278.

Greenley, James R. "Family Symptom Tolerance and Rehospitalization Experiences of Psychiatric Patients," in Roberta Simmons, ed., *Research in Community and Mental Health.* Greenwich, Conn.: Jai Press, 1979. Pp. 357-386.

Gruenberg, Ernest. "Hospital Treatment in Schizophrenia," in Robert Cancro, ed., *The Schizophrenic Reactions: A Critique of the Concept, Hospital Treatment, and Current Research.* New York: Brunner/Mazel, 1970.

Hoenig, Julius, and Hamilton, Marian W. *The Desegregation of the Mentally Ill.* London, England: Routledge & Kegan Paul, 1969.

Hollingshead, August B., and Redlich, Frederick C. *Social Class and Mental Illness.* New York: John Wiley & Sons. 1958.

Kellum, Sheppard G.; Ensminger, Margaret E.; and Turner, Jay. "Family Structure and the Mental Health of Children," *Archives of General Psychiatry,* 34 (September 1977), pp. 1012-1022.

Kreisman, Dolores E., and Joy, Virginia D. "Family Response to the Mental Illness of a Relative: A Literature Review," *Schizophrenia Bulletin,* 10 (Fall 1974), pp. 35-55.

Michaux, William W. et al: *The First Year Out.* Baltimore, Md.: Johns Hopkins University Press, 1969.

Miller, Dorothea. *Worlds that Fail, Part I: Retrospective Analysis of Mental Patients' Careers.* Sacramento, Calif.: California State Department of Mental Hygiene, 1965.

Mills, E. *Living with Mental Illness: A Study of East London.* London, England: Routledge & Kegan Paul, 1962.

Myers, Jerome K., and Bean, Lee L. *A Decade Later: A Follow-up of Social Class and Mental Illness.* New York: John Wiley & Sons, 1968.

Myers, Jerome K., and Roberts, Bertram H. *Family and Class Dynamics in Mental Illness.* New York: John Wiley & Sons, 1959.

Pasamanick, Benjamin; Scarpitti, Frank R.; and Dinitz, Simon. *Schizophrenics in the Community.* New York: Appleton-Century-Crofts, 1967.

Phillips, Derek L. "Rejection: A Possible Consequence of Seeking Help for Mental Disorders," *American Sociological Review,* 28 (December 1963), pp. 962-963.

Pitt, Raymond. "The Concept of Family Burden." Unpublished manuscript, Columbia University, 1960.

Rawnsley, K.; Loudon, J. B.; and Miles, H. L. "Attitudes of Relatives to Patients in Mental Hospitals," *British Journal of Preventive and Social Medicine,* 16 (January 1962), pp. 1-15.

Robins, Lee N. *Deviant Children Grown Up: A Sociological and Psychiatric Study of Sociopathic Personality.* Baltimore, Md.: Williams & Wilkins, 1966. P. 174.

Rogler, Lloyd H., and Hollingshead, August. *Trapped: Families and Schizophrenia.* New York: John Wiley & Sons, 1965.

Rose, Charles L. "Relatives' Attitudes and Mental Hospitalization," *Mental Hygiene*, 43 (April 1959), pp. 194-203.

Schwartz, Carol; Myers, Jerome K.; and Astrachan, Boris M. "Psychiatric Labeling and the Rehabilitation of the Mental Patient," *Archives of General Psychiatry*, 31 (September 1974), pp. 329-334.

Segal, Steven P. "Preventing Social Deterioration in Former Mental Patients." Paper presented at the National Conference on Social Welfare, Los Angeles, Calif., May 1978.

Segal, Steven P., and Aviram, Uri. "Community-Based Sheltered Care," in Paul I. Ahmed and Stanley C. Plog, eds., *State Mental Hospitals: What Happens When They Close?* New York: Plenum Publishing Corp., 1976. Pp. 111-124.

————. *The Mentally Ill in Community-Based Sheltered Care.* New York: Wiley Inter-Science, 1978.

Segal, Steven P., and Moyles, Edwin W. "Management Style and Institutional Dependency in Sheltered Care." To be published in a forthcoming issue of *Social Psychiarty*.

Sommer, Robert. "Letter-Writing in a Mental Hospital," *American Journal of Psychiatry*, 115 (December 1958), pp. 518-519.

————. "Visitors to Mental Hospitals: A Fertile Field for Research," *Mental Hygiene*, 43 (January 1959), pp. 8-15.

Stein, Leonard I.; Test, Mary Ann; and Marx, Arnold J. "Alternative to the Hospital: A Controlled Study," *American Journal of Psychiatry*, 132 (May 1975), pp. 517-532.

Swanson, Robert M., and Spitzer, Stephen P. "Stigma and the Psychiatric Patient Career," *Journal of Health and Social Behavior*, 11 (March 1970), pp. 44-51.

Swingle, Paul G. "Relatives' Concepts of Mental Patients," *Mental Hygiene*, 49 (July 1965), pp. 461-465.

Wing, John; Monck, Elizabeth; Brown, George; and Carstairs, G. M. "Morbidity in the Community of Schizophrenic Patients Discharged from London Mental Hospitals in 1959," *British Journal of Psychiatry*, 110 (January 1964), pp. 10-21.

# Family Supports in Old Age

## Abraham Monk

The last two decades have produced an astounding record of legislative advances on behalf of the aged. A relentless flurry of political activism and public policymaking began to steamroll in 1959, immediately after the creation of the Senate's Special Committee on Aging. Some of the changes included the following:

1. The Medicare and Medicaid amendments to the Social Security Act;
2. The Older Americans Act, which was signed into law in 1965 to foster planning and development of services for the elderly at the local level;
3. The Age Discrimination Act of 1967;
4. The 1975 Comprehensive Service amendments to the Older Americans Act;
5. The 1974 Supplemental Security Income amendments to the Social Security Act;
6. A major reform bill for pensions; and
7. A cost-of-living clause escalating social security benefits.

The aged succeeded in heightening their political visibility, and in the process, they outdistanced other interest groups and political movements in net gains in social policy. The sociological debate on whether the aged emerged as a subculture, a minority, or a mere demographic cohort is rather inconsequential. What matters is that the political activity of the aged and their advocates was far more effective than the politicking of other claimants in the political arena.

Aging as a cause is not a temporary fad endorsed by a marginal following. The elderly constitute nearly 25 percent of the voters, and they have a remarkable capacity for mobilization. It would be misleading, however, to attribute their effectiveness to the sheer weight of numbers. Aging seems to touch a deeper emotional cord among legislators. For some, it conjures images and afflictions of their ailing parents; for others it may project personal concerns about impending senescence. In any event, political sympathies for the aged were so overwhelming in the early seventies that some congressional actions such as the increase in social security benefits in 1972—and the concomitant increase in social security taxes for current wage earners—were passed regardless of the symptoms of discontent beginning among taxpayers. Moreover, two years later, Congress did not hesitate to vote a further 11 percent boost in social security benefits, even when it was apparent that the costs were far from negligible.

Federal spending on behalf of the aged precipitiously increased from 25 billion dollars in fiscal year (FY) 1967 to 229 billion dollars in FY 1972. Benefits related to aging, which represented 15.8 percent of the total federal budget in 1967, expanded to 20.2 percent of the budget in 1972 and continued to escalate until they were 24 percent in FY 1978.[1] Programs for the aged will claim an even greater share of federal dollars if present trends in financing continue, and the aged may well require 40 percent of the total federal outlay by 2010, when the "baby boom" of the 1940s and 1950s turns into a critical "senior boom."[2]

## DEMOGRAPHIC TRENDS

Social policy is affected by changes in the composition of age groups. It is affected also by changes in residential patterns of families. The following three salient demographic and ecological characteristics are particularly important and need to be underscored.[3]

1. *People are living increasingly longer.* In 1900, life expectancy at birth was 48.2 for white males and 51.1 for females. For blacks it was 32.5 and 35 for men and women, respectively. In 1974, it rose to 68.0 and 76.6 for white men and women and 62.9 and 71.2 for black men and women, a virtual doubling of the average life expectancy for the latter group. The proportion of older persons relative to the total population is also increasing. In 1900, the age group of 65 and older constituted less than 4 percent of the population, and projections show that this group will more than

triple proportionately by the year 2000, reaching the 14 percent mark or one in every seven Americans.

2. *The older population is predominantly female.* Because women outlive men, the present ratio is 70 males to 100 females in the age group of 65 and older. But at age 75, the imbalance is even more pronounced—58 males for every 100 females.

3. *Most elderly men live with their spouse.* As a corollary of the above, nearly 75 percent of the elderly males lived in a household with a spouse present, compared with nearly 40 percent of women in the same age bracket. Because women enjoy a higher life expectancy, they frequently become widowed while men often remain married until they die. Eighty percent of older men are married; sixty-one percent of elderly women are widowed. These figures also reflect that fact that elderly widowers are seven times more likely to remarry than are comparably aged widows. Moreover, 36 percent of the women and only 14 percent of the men live in single-person households. These figures show a substantial departure from the residential pattern older women, in particular, experienced in earlier decades—that is, they no longer live with someone else, usually a daughter, but live alone. Old men are even less likely to be living in the home of an adult child.

The policy implications of these facts are clear. Given the longer life expectancy, morbidity rates inevitably go up. The number of multiproblem, frail elderly—actually the most intensive consumers of health and social services—is increasing at a faster rate than the overall number of elderly. Many critical problems of old age such as low income, loneliness, and poor health are rooted in the overrepresentation of widowed and nonmarried females.

Longer life expectancy means adding more generations to family networks too. The four-generation family is no longer a rarity. It would be precipitous and unfounded, however, to assume the advent of the neo-extended family. There is no evidence yet that the neo-extended family is a viable unit in circumstances other than emergencies such as bereavement, acute illness, and disasters. Grandparents may be losing ground even in three-generation families. Kahana and Kahana and Wood and Robertson found that although grandchildren harbor positive attitudes toward their grandparents, they do not assign them a central role in their lives.[4] Grandparents are not chosen as companions, advisors, or role models by their grandchildren.

## INTERGENERATIONAL INCOME TRANSFERS

Social policies have moved away from the Elizabethan Poor Law, which established that the community would assist an indigent parent only after the means of the child had been called on. Until very recently, the majority of states kept statutory provisions in their public assistance laws prescribing the obligation adult children had toward the financial support of their parents. In practice, attempts to enforce filial support under those public assistance laws did not work or were administratively too cumbersome. Burr found that costs involved in such collections often exceeded the actual payments extracted from reluctant children.[5] Schorr added that enforcement of filial responsibility brought about detrimental effects to all parties concerned. Enforcement perpetuated poverty because children could seldom attend to their parents' needs without jeopardizing the support of their own progeny, it generated feelings of guilt among the aged, and it prevented middle-aged children from saving for their own old age.[6]

Filial-responsibility clauses have faded from legislation enacted in the last fifteen years. Yet massive intergenerational transfers do occur albeit indirectly and disguised as social insurance in our social security program. As stated by Gold, the federal government intervenes on behalf of the aged through six concurrent roles: income maintenance; noncash benefits with measurable economic value such as health care financing; protection of rights; research; financial support for social services in the public and voluntary sectors; and coordination and "orchestration" of the preceding five roles.[7] Income maintenance, with social security as its major component, is the primary stratagem and is by far more important than all other types of intervention combined. Income maintenance programs are intended to enhance individual independence and reduce filial responsibility. Without them, nearly 60 percent of the elderly family units would have fallen below the poverty line in 1976.[8]

Nobody has ventured to formally propose a fourth option, that is, to dismantle the social security system and expect filial responsibility to take over. There is no chance that the current generation of workers would lay out 100 billion dollars a year from their own pockets to support their retired parents. Indeed, the essence of the income maintenance strategy for the aged that has evolved since passage of the Social Security Act in 1935 has been geared toward neutralizing the risks of parental dependency on children. The strategy affirms that family ties are no longer economic and that children have no legal responsibility to support their aging parents. The law acknowledges that the culture of the United States emphasizes personal freedom, which seems to imply that many people think becoming dependent is a sign of having "failed" in life. The "I'd rather die than ask my children for help" syndrome does not do justice, however, to the extensive assistance that adult children provide their elders. Moreover, that this assistance is often made at the cost of substantial sacrifices in the lives of adult children has been empirically determined in studies by Shanas, Bell, and Cantor.[9]

## *ROLE STRAIN*

Regardless of the extent to which families do support elderly members, the myth of "family abandonment" continues to exist. Brody alludes to this pervasive myth, which says that helpless, older parents are ignored by their insensitive offspring.[10] She states that the myth may reflect the guilt of a youth-oriented society seeking to rationalize its lack of abeyance to the "etiquette of filial behavior," that is, the deference to elders practiced by youth in past years and in more traditional societies. Brody lists multiple determinants that feed the myth and keep it alive. She mentions, for example, that professional service workers who are frequently in touch with a biased sample of older persons—that is, those older persons who are childless or alienated from their children—often assume that this bias actually reflects universal patterns of intergenerational relationships.

Although the myth of family abandonment is unfair to adult children, role conflicts are bound to occur. Filial responsibilities, for example, often impinge on the quality of a husband-wife relationship. Goode analyzed the "role strain" resulting from concurrent demands on beleaguered individuals with multiple roles to fill.[11] Adult children have a sense of obligation toward their aging parents because of the time and effort their parents invested in them during their growth and development. However, Streib's research on retired fathers and their adult offspring suggests that when faced with the crucial dilemma of choosing between their own children and spouses or their aging parents, the adult offspring tend to choose in favor of the former.[12] In addition, as is often observed in practice with families of the aged, willingness to help aging parents is not always a valid indicator of the ability or actual readiness to provide such help on a continuous basis. Parsons and Fox have suggested that the emotional balance of the American family is seriously jeopardized by the imposition of disability or chronic, prolonged illness and that good relations often deteriorate in face of the added burden.[13]

Role strain not only affects adult children but also affects each member of an elderly couple. This principle of independence rather than interdependence in income-related matters, for example, is being legally affirmed not only for children but also for spouses. Until recently Medicaid was denied to a sick older adult until his or her spouse had exhausted almost all personal resources. A fair hearing in New York State handed down on April 17, 1979 found that the State Department of Social Services could not deny assistance to a wife, age 77, who was in a nursing home when her husband refused to continue payments. The husband, also age 77, had some resources left but after paying $36,700, felt he should not become impoverished since, by law, the state was required to pay for her care. Following the hearing, the department ruled that the resources and income of spouses over age 65 should be treated separately after six months of physical separation. The ruling stated that after institutionalization of one spouse for at least six months, the spouse at home would no longer be reduced to poverty level in order for Medicaid to pay the nursing costs. The spouse at home could retain some assets and income, and couples married 40 or 50 years would no longer have to resort to divorce.[14]

## BARRIERS TO CARE

Although the principles of intergenerational separation and independence seem firmly established by law in the domain of income maintenance, substantial ambiguity and confusion still remain as to the family's role in the provision of health care, one of the most pressing needs elderly people experience. That the aged use health services three times more often than the rest of the population will come as no surprise to human services providers. However, what needs to be underscored, in particular, is that in the next 50 years, health costs for the aged will increase by a factor of ten—a statistic that will exceed the increase in social security benefits by two.[15] Because health costs threaten to exceed an individual's capacity to pay, whether by governmental subsidy or by private income, the health system will have to rely less on hospitalization and institutionalization and will have to focus instead on home health care for both acute and chronic illnesses of the aged. Tax rebates, cash allotments, and community support could provide incentives for families who would care for their aged at home. In fact, the initiative to expand home health services is actually predicated on the expectation that informal support networks of relatives, friends, and neighbors will be revitalized and will assume more explicit, if only supplemental, caregiving roles. If this does not occur, the formal health system by itself will be unable to contend with such a large and expanding population at risk as the aged. If reliance on the availability of family support systems becomes excessive, however, undesirable policy consequences may result.

It is argued, for instance, that the skyrocketing costs of longterm care for the aged and the alleged failures of the Medicaid program to contain nursing home costs could be handled if children and other relatives accepted more responsibility for the care of their elderly members. The assumption, however, that institutional care ultimately may be phased out or reduced and that potentially families will be capable of taking care of their elderly members overlooks a few essential facts. First, the institutionalized elderly population has a mean age of 82, with over 70 percent of the group exceeding age 70. Most members of this population are women, including widows and a sizeable segment of single, never-married women. Almost half do not have close relatives, and many widows have outlived their own children.[16]

Second, it has been estimated that families already provide as much as 80 percent of home health care services for older relatives.[17] Families fill the gaps and deficiencies of the service system, they contend with the bewildering maze of entitlements, and they advocate for the aged in relentless negotiations with public bureaucracies. Families also shop for the aged, escort them on trips, help them with household chores, and even attend courses that will enable them to undertake complex rehabilitative care functions. Policymakers wonder, however, how much maintenance a family can provide beyond essential chores and socioemotional supports. Is there an erosion with time of such capacity, and if so, what kind of program could assist the family to increase its effectiveness in caretaking? In any event, policymakers cannot deny that family ties, no matter how close, do not have a legal, binding quality but remain essentially voluntary.

Third, there are, of course, many types of families. They vary in terms of their internal cohesion and unconditional availability. In addition, generations are becoming geographically separated. In 1957, of those persons 65 years of age and older who had children, 36 percent lived with one child. Less than twenty years later, in 1975, that percentage had shrunk in half to 18 percent.[18] Relatives still support and care for aged family members at home, but geographic separation adds one more barrier to the possibility of this option. Health programs aimed at enhancing the mutuality between formal and informal systems will, therefore, have to recognize the fact that families will be less available as providers of traditional and concrete services.

Fourth, declining fertility rates today will mean fewer descendents for aging parents to call on in crises. Finally, new roles assumed by women in the job market will reduce their availability to perform traditional caregiving roles.

## *NONTRADITIONAL CARE*

In essence, the aged will need a greater array of health services, regardless of the availability of primary support networks, ranging from comprehensive long-term care to home delivered services. These will include day care, respite care, semi-independent sheltered housing and foster care, and protective services. In the absence of support networks, appropriate surrogates such as peer support and self-help networks should be encouraged. Living arrangements such as age-segregated housing and communal associations are being seen with more favor.

Resistance toward age-segregated housing is still common, however, among social workers despite research findings that consistently show such housing, when voluntarily chosen, produces positive feelings of personal security for the elderly as well as increased morale and informal social interactions. Regardless of this resistance, people in many areas of the United States are experimenting with models of communal and cooperative living arrangements. The "Share-A-Home" program, for example, started in Florida in 1972 and provides cooperative family living for ambulatory, nonrelated senior persons who live together in a home, eat together, and share birthdays, outings, and celebrations. A manager and staff are hired to care for their housekeeping needs, finances, laundry, and transportation.[19] This experiment aims to overcome the gaps in living arrangements and social interactions that elderly people experience when real families can longer provide support. Another example of this type of care is the Jewish Federation of Metropolitan Chicago, which has a stronger infusion of social services, including a full-time caseworker and a psychiatrist who is on call.[20]

It is too early to predict whether these experimental communities will be adopted widely and, ultimately if they will prove to be effective. These models do recognize one important fact, however. It is that euphoric expectations about primary support networks are not justified. Families do not possess unending resources for attending to the complex health and social needs of their aging relatives. Planners in these communities realize that comprehensive systems of health and social services should be meshed with parallel supports, including new models of surrogate family and communal associations in addition to the more traditional family networks.

## NOTES AND REFERENCES

1. Unpublished statistics, estimated by the Social Security Administration. April 1978, as cited in Joseph A. Califano, Jr., "The Aging of America: Questions for the Four Generation Society," *Annals of the American Academy of Political and Social Science,* 438 (July 1978), p. 98.

2. Ibid., p. 99

3. U.S. Bureau of the Census, "Demographic Aspects of Aging and the Older Population in the United States," *Current Population Reports,* Series P-23, No. 43 (February 1973), p. 23, and Series P-23, No. 59 (May 1976), p. 8.

4. Eva Kahana and Boaz Kahana, "Theoretical and Research Perspectives of Grandparenthood," *Aging and Human Development,* 2. No. 4 (1971), pp. 261-268; and Vivian Wood and Joan Robertson, "The Significance of Grandparenthood," in Jaber Gubrium, ed., *Times, Roles and Self in Old Age* (New York: Human Sciences Press, 1976).

5. James J. Burr, "Financial Support of the Aged By Their Relatives," *Living in the Multigenerational Family,* "Occasional Papers in Gerontology," Vol. 3 (Ann Arbor: Institute of Gerontology, The University of Michigan, 1969), pp. 60-77.

6. Alvin L. Schorr, *Filial Responsibility in the Modern American Family* (Washington, D.C.: Social Security Administration, Division of Program Research, Department of Health, Education & Welfare, 1960), pp. 27-31.

7. Byron D. Gold, "The Role of the Federal Government in the Provision of Social Services to Older Persons," *Annals of the American Academy of Political and Social Science,* 415 (September 1974), pp. 55-69.

8. U.S. Bureau of the Census, "Money Income and Poverty Status of Families and Persons in the United States: 1976," *Current Population Reports,* Series P-60, No. 107 (September 1977), p. 60.

9. Ethel Shanas, "Family-Kin Networks and Aging in Cross Cultural Perspective," *Journal of Marriage and The Family,* 35 (August 1973), pp. 505-511; William G. Bell, "Filial Responsibility, Social Provision and Social Policy: A Study of Their Relationship," unpublished doctoral thesis, Brandeis University, 1969; and Marjorie Cantor, "Life Space

and the Social Support System of the Inner City Elderly of New York," *Gerontologist,* 15 (1975), pp. 15, 23-27.

10. Elaine M. Brody, "Serving the Aged: Educational Needs As Viewed by Practice," *Social Work,* 15 (October 1970), p. 42.

11. William J. Goode, "A Theory of Role Strain," *American Sociological Review,* 25 (August 1960), pp. 483-496.

12. Gordon F. Streib, "Integenerational Relations: Perspectives of the Two Generation Family on the Older Parent," *Journal of Marriage and the Family,* 27 (November 1965), pp. 469-476.

13. Talcott Parsons and Renée Fox, "Illness, Therapy and the Modern Urban Family," *Journal of Social Issues,* 8, No. 4 (1952), pp. 31-44.

14. Press release, Brookdale Center on Aging, Hunter College, New York, New York, June 8, 1979, p. 2.

15. Unpublished statistics calculated by the Social Security Administration, April 1978, as cited in Califano, op. cit.

16. Subcommittee on Long-Term Care, *Nursing Home Care in the United States: Failure in Public Policy,* Report to U.S. Senate Special Committee on Aging, Publication No. 40-057-0 (Washington, D.C.: U.S. Government Printing Office, 1974), p. 16.

17. National Center for Health Statistics, U.S. Department of Health, Education and Welfare, "Home Health Care for Persons 55 Years and Over," *Vital and Health Statistics Publication Statistics Publication Series,* 10, No. 73 (1972), p. 2.

18. Ethel Shanas, *Health of Older People: A Social Survey* (Cambridge, Mass.: Harvard University Press, 1962), p. 96; and unpublished data from *National Sample Survey of Institutional Persons 65 Years of Age and Older in the U.S., 1975,* funded by the Social Security Administration (Washington, D.C.: U.S. Department of Health, Education & Welfare, u.d.) (Mimeographed).

19. Gordon F. Streib, "An Alternative Family Form For Older Persons: Need and Social Context." *The Family Coordinator,* 27 (October 1978), pp. 413-420.

20. J. Wax, "It's Like Your Own Home Here," *New York Times Magazine,* November 21, 1976, p. 38.

# Adolescent Mothers and Their Children: Another Population that Requires Family Care

Lorraine V. Klerman

When Americans think of the three generation household, they usually perceive it as comprising grandparents reaching the end of their life cycles, parents in their most productive years, and their children who have not yet reached adulthood. Television's Walton family exemplifies such a household. Historical studies of the family now suggest that this type of household actually has been relatively uncommon in America (Smith, 1979). Another type of three generation household, however, is apparently increasing in prevalence. It consists of grandparents still in their most productive years, their children including an unmarried female adolescent, and her young infant. This article will review the new patterns of adolescent and adult behavior which have resulted in this trend as well as the supports that are necessary if the adolescent is to accomplish her difficult dual tasks of personal maturation and child rearing, if her child is to develop maximally, and if the adult generation is not to be unduly penalized.

## ADOLESCENT PARENTING—
## ITS EMERGENCE AS A PROBLEM

The emergence of adolescent parenting as a social welfare problem is relatively recent. Child rearing by youth under age twenty was not considered inappropriate in earlier civilizations or even in America prior to the 1960s, so long as it occurred within marriage. Illegitimacy was the behavior to be avoided regardless of age.

The assistance in the preparation of this chapter of Jacob Alex Klerman, E. Milling Kinard, and Fern Marx is gratefully acknowledged.

*111*

While it is undoubtedly true that a large portion of the current negative reaction to adolescent child rearing is caused by the high proportion of illegitimate births and/or conceptions in this age group, several trends have influenced the shift to an age-related concern.

## Prolongation of Adolescence

The first important trend is the prolongation of the adolescent years—some say the creation of the adolescent period. As industrial societies have become increasingly complex, the period needed to prepare for adult work roles has increased. Graduation from high school has become essential for obtaining employment which can generate wages sufficient to support a family. Entry into the labor force today occurs later than it did in previous generations. Coleman (1974) has noted, "As the labor of children has become unnecessary to society, school has been extended for them. With every decade, the length of school has increased, until a thoughtful person must ask whether society can conceive of no other way for youth to come into adulthood."

## Increase in Sexual Activity

Unfortunately, the prolongation of the period of economic dependence has not been accompanied by an absence of sexual interest or activity. To the contrary, both biological and social factors have conspired to make the trials of adolescence more difficult. The age of sexual maturity gradually has declined until current studies suggest that on the average females are fertile by age 14 and males by age 15.5 (Rauh et al., 1973). Further complicating the situation has been a documented increase in sexual activity among teenage females. It is currently estimated that 69 percent of never-married women have experienced intercourse by age 19.*

---

*Zelnik and Kantner (1980) found that between their 1971 and 1979 national surveys of 15-19 year old women, sexual activity for never-married whites had increased 82 percent and for never-married blacks 24 percent. By 1979, at age 15, 18 percent of never-married whites as compared to 41 percent of never-married blacks had engaged in intercourse and by age 19, the rates were 65 percent for whites and 89 percent for blacks.

## Rise in Adolescent Births

This increase in sexual activity began at a time when the number of adolescent females at risk for pregnancy was high as a result of the large cohort of post-World War II infants reaching the fertile years (Newsweek, 1981). Consequently the number of births to all teenagers reached over six hundred and fifty thousand in 1970 and to adolescents 17 and under, over two hundred and fifty thousand in 1973. Although the numbers themselves were alarming, the concern among health, education, and social service agencies, as well as the general public, was heightened by several factors: (1) the documentation of the increased medical risks to mothers and infants, as well as the negative social consequences associated with early childbearing; (2) the decline in fertility among older women which caused teenage births to become a larger percentage of all births; (3) an increase in births to the very young (under age 15) to over twelve thousand from 1972 to 1975; and (4) a rise in the percentage of teenage births that were illegitimate. Fortunately the latter part of the 1970s witnessed a decline in both the number and the rate of births to females under 20.* The downward trend is encouraging, but clearly a problem of major dimensions still exists.

## Changes in Societal Response

The premaritally pregnant adolescent has several choices available: marriage, adoption, abortion, or single parenthood. Adolescent childbearing might not be increasing the number of individuals dependent on the family for care and support if changes had not occurred in societal attitudes toward these alternatives.

*Marriage:* Today's adolescents appear less convinced that marriage is a necessary condition for childbearing—and, equally puzzling, seem to believe that marriage requires more maturity and commitment than having a child. Today's adults appear more accepting of youthful parenting, even outside of marriage. Prior to the 1960s, among white populations at least, one traditional

---

*In 1978 there were over 554 thousand births to women 12-19 years of age and over 213 thousand to adolescents 17 and under. The birth rates per thousand women were 1.2 for 10-14 year olds, 32.9 for 15-17 year olds, and 81.0 for 18-19 year olds, down from 1.3 for 10-14s in 1975, from 39.2 for 15-17s in 1972, and from over 120 for 18-19s before 1970 (Centers for Disease Control, 1981 and Public Health Service, 1981).

response to adolescent pregnancy in an unmarried adolescent was a "shotgun marriage." A young woman who "got into trouble" often was expected to reveal the name of her male partner and he was forced to "make an honest woman of her." These phrases seem antiquated—one seldom hears them today and as a consequence, illegitimate births to teenagers have increased. Nevertheless, post-conception marriages still occur. O'Connell and Moore (1980) estimated that in the 1971-74 period, 65 percent of the 15-19 year old but only 53 percent of the 15-17 old white women who were premaritally pregnant married before the birth of their first child, and among 15-19 year old blacks the rate was 17 percent.* In 1978, however, 57.5 percent of all live births to 15-17 year old women were to unmarried women (Public Health Service, 1981).

The present separation between marriage and parenting has been noted by several researchers who quote their pregnant respondents as stating that they were not ready for marriage, although they planned to bear and rear their children. Grandmothers seem to share this attitude. Furstenberg (1980a) reported that an interviewer was told concerning marriage:

> She'll have enough time for that. I want her to stay in school so she won't have to be dependent when she grows up. She can stay with us until she completes her education.

Furstenberg's sample was predominantly black, but a commentator on the white population made a similar observation. Trudeau (1980) in a Doonesbury cartoon has two young people talking to the female's mother:

> We know you think we should wait, that marriage is a big commitment, and that we shouldn't rush into it the way you did. Well, we agree with you now . . . Yes. So we've decided to postpone the wedding until we figure out what we're going to do with our lives . . . (Relieved mother: "Well dear, I think that's a very mature . . . ") We're still going to go ahead with the kid, though . . . Right. While we're still young enough to enjoy him.

---

*These percentages were down from 76 percent for 15-19 year old and 73 percent for 15-17 year old white women in 1955-1958 and from 37 percent for 15-19 year old black women in the 1947-1950 period.

*Adoption:* The usual alternative to a post-conception marriage among whites has been adoption. The pregnant adolescent was sent to a maternity home or to a relative in a distant city where she delivered the infant and gave it up for adoption. She then returned home to pick up her life as if nothing had happened—in fact, as few individuals as possible were informed of what had transpired. Such a solution to the problem of adolescent pregnancy is not longer used by the vast proportion of pregnant adolescents. This has been documented not only by interviews with adolescents (Zelnik and Kantner, 1978), but also by the decline both in the number of infants available for adoption and in the number of maternity homes and women served by them (Wallace et al., 1974).

*Abortion:* If neither marriage nor adoption are currently acceptable to a large percentage of pregnant adolescents, the remaining alternatives are abortion and single parenthood. Many choose abortion.\* The increase in the number of abortions and the decrease in the number of adoptions suggests that pregnant adolescents who do not want to care for an infant opt for abortions.

## SINGLE PARENTHOOD

For the adolescent mother who chooses single parenthood, several alternative living arrangements are theoretically available. She and her infant may live alone, with other unrelated females or males, with her parents, with other relatives, in a foster home, or in a group facility. Her decision will be influenced by her preferences (Gorbach and Messenger, 1982), the feelings of her parents or other relatives, and by her needs for a variety of types of assistance.

### Alternative Living Arrangements

*Independent households:* Despite the potential problems of loneliness and the absence of social supports, some young mothers decide to establish independent households after delivery or a year or two later. The most common reasons given, according to welfare

---

\*In 1978 the estimated number of legal abortions was over eighteen thousand among females 12-14, over 196 thousand among 15-17 year olds, and over 244 thousand among 18 and 19 year olds. The abortion ratios were 617 legal abortions per 1000 births among white famales 14 and under and 629 among blacks; 665 and 620 for white and black 15-17 year olds; and 581 and 668 for white and black 18 and 19 year olds. (Ezzard et al., 1982).

staff and caseworkers, is family strife, including anger about the pregnancy and conflicts over the raising of the infant, with the adolescent mother claiming her mother is assuming too much responsibility—a "whose child is this?" situation.

Workers also suspect that the decision often is influenced by basic adolescent independence issues even when they are not explicit. Although the vast majority of adolescent births are unplanned, the decision not to abort, as well as other indicators, suggest that many of the infants are not unwanted. For the adolescent, particularly the low income adolescent or the one with low self-esteem, the birth of a baby and the assumption of care-taking responsibilities are ways of proving her self-worth. These events may increase her desire to remove herself from two settings where she may have felt dependent and perhaps inadequate—home and school. It is not surprising, therefore, that many adolescents at least explore the possibilities of leaving their families. They generally have unrealistic images about the glamour of an apartment of their own, but very correct impressions of how easy it would be to drop out of school in the absence of parental encouragement, supervision, and child care.

For some young mothers, life in an independent household, foster placement, or a group facility is not a matter of choice, but is forced upon them. Some parents cannot face the prospect of life with an unmarried adolescent daughter who is pregnant or who is a mother caring for her child. Such a family may push the daughter out of its household soon after the pregnancy is announced or after the infant is born. The number of young mothers living independently also is increased by the few who never tell their parents of their pregnancies, but instead run away from home in fear of what would happen if their parents discovered their condition.

*With a family:* The few, small studies of the living arrangements of adolescent parents indicate that a very small number of mother-infant pairs are in foster care or group settings, that some live separate from their parents or other relatives, but that most reside with a family, usually parents but occasionally aunts, sisters, or other relatives. The incorporation of the young mother and her child into the parental household, as well as the decline in marriage and adoption, suggests a major change in the attitudes toward single parenthood among American families. With varying degrees of pain and discomfort many white families are accepting the pregnancies of their daughters and their decisions to bear and raise a child outside of marriage. An article in *MS* magazine entitled "Teenage Mothers are Keeping Their Babies—with the Help of Their Own Mothers" (Leishman, 1980) featured a white teenager, her baby, and her mother. The mother is quoted as saying:

> Well, she wanted to keep the baby—none of us believes in abortion—and she didn't want to get married which was okay with us. After all, fifteen is kind of young to marry, and we wanted her to finish high school and go to college. Anyway, I've had ten kids, so as long as I can remember there's always been a baby in the house, and this one is our pride and joy.

Some black families had adopted this three generation household pattern earlier. The younger initiation of sexual activity, the absence of a black adoption market, less availability of family planning and abortion services, and high teenage unemployment made adolescent childbearing more prevalent and alternatives to single parenthood less feasible in this minority group. In a follow-up study of almost four hundred predominantly black females under 18 who sought prenatal care at Sinai Hospital in Baltimore in 1966-1967, Furstenberg and Crawford (1978) found that approximately one year after delivery, 77 percent of the married and unmarried respondents lived in their parents' or relatives' homes. Although 36 percent of all respondents had been married and 28 percent were currently married, 43 percent of the currently married were still living with parents or kin (usually the woman's). Seven percent of all respondents were living alone and the remainder (16 percent) with spouse only. Two years later, when the children were three and the mothers in their late teens or early twenties, 63 percent of the entire sample continued to live with one or both parents or other relatives. Now 52 percent had been married, 36 percent were currently married, and 31 percent of the currently married still were living with parents or kin. Only 12 percent of all respondents had established independent households and 25 percent lived with spouse only. At the final interview five years after the child's birth, 46 percent were living with their families. Sixty-three percent had been married, 33 percent were currently married, and 18 percent of the currently married were still living with parents or kin. Twenty-six percent of the respondents were living alone and 27 percent with a spouse only.

Although the pattern probably still is more frequent among black families, apparently now both races often allow the young woman to stay in her family's home during the pregnancy and to return there with her infant after delivery. Thus a three-generation household is created which may last a few months or a few years depending on the age of the new mother and the accommodations reached between her and her mother, principally, but with other household members as well.

### Needs of Mother and Infant

Regardless of living arrangements, the pregnant adolescent or young mother has many needs, including medical care, educational services, income, day care, counseling, and assistance in learning how to be a parent—as well as food and shelter. Her infant also requires food and shelter, plus medical care and social stimulation. This wide variety of often urgent needs provides a rationale for many parents and relatives to urge unmarried adolescents to live with them, but also suggests why some families are reluctant to assume the burden.

If the adolescent mother and her child stay with her parents or other relatives, they are almost certainly going to make demands on that unit. One such demand will be for space. An infant may only require a crib, but if its feeding schedule and other needs are not to interfere with other household functions and its sleep is not to be disturbed by those functions, the crib should be placed in a separate room or one which is not in continual use. Toddlers may no longer need separate sleeping quarters, but their curiosity may cause them to venture frequently into space claimed by others.

Infants and toddlers also make demands on time. Although the young mother should assume major responsibility for the care of her child, there will be times when she requests help from family members. Particularly if she returns to school, she may need others to feed, diaper, amuse, and in other ways spend time with her child. Even if she has completed school or dropped out, the young mother will often want to spend time with friends and ask others to baby-sit. Since most communities have a shortage of day care slots, particularly infant day care places, it is often the grandmother who will be expected to care for the child. If the grandmother worked prior to the birth of the infant, she may not wish to relinquish her job in order to provide child care, but arrangements with siblings, other relatives, or babysitters often are unreliable and not conducive to the physical and/or emotional health of the infant.

Privacy and quiet are other precious commodities in many households. The presence of an infant or toddler frequently places these items in scarce supply. Adolescent mothers often report that tempers flare when an infant cries in the middle of the night or a toddler interferes with a favorite television program.

Of equal or greater importance, however, is the strain on economic resources. The economic needs of the adolescent daughter continue and may even increase, and added to these are the child's need for food, clothing, furniture, and medical care. The child's father and/or his family may contribute to its upkeep and in almost all states the infant is eligible for funds from Aid to Families with Dependent Children (AFDC) and Medicaid, but these sources seldom cover all the additional expenses incurred by the mother-infant unit.

Thus there are many good reasons why parents or other relatives may have mixed feelings about the prospect of incorporating the new mother and her infant into their households. The alternative living arrangements, however, often provide fewer of the financial, emotional, and other resources needed by mother and child.

## *Benefits of Family Care*

While the isolated mother and child in an independent household may have food, shelter, and medical care provided by AFDC and Medicaid, the absence of other individuals, particularly adults, may have negative consequences. The young mother in such a setting usually drops out of school because of problems finding day care for her child and the lack of parental encouragement. The absence of parental supervision may also make easier both sexual activity and contraceptive neglect, leading to a rapid subsequent pregnancy.

Also, the young mother's inability to leave the house to attend school or to spend time with friends and the absence of anyone with whom to share the burdens of child rearing may cause frustration and lead to withdrawn or aggressive behavior. As a result, the infant may suffer, if not because of actual abuse perhaps through neglect or inadequate parenting (Kinard and Klerman, 1980; Leventhal, 1981).

In addition, young mothers may be unaware of the needs of infants beyond physical care. Current research stresses the importance of physical contact, verbalization, visual stimulation, play, and many other adult-infant interactions. The young mother living with adult relatives may learn these activities by observing and meanwhile the infant will benefit from its contacts with other adults. The infant living with its mother alone may have fewer of these experiences which are so important to its normal development.

The findings of several research studies support the concept that family care is beneficial for both mother and child. For example, Furstenberg and Crawford (1978) in their five-year follow-up study found that among the 36 percent of the study population who never married, those who remained with their parents or kin as compared to those who were living alone were more likely to have returned to school (87%-76%), completed high school (62%-47%), and been employed (60%-41%), and were less likely to be on welfare (43%-65%). For women who married and subsequently separated few differences were found between women who returned to live with their parents and women who set up independent households. Neither of the latter groups fared as well on the socioeconomic indicators as the never-married living with parents. Women who remained married and lived with their husbands achieved the lowest level of welfare dependence of any of the groups (12%) and did better than the other never-married groups on some of the indicators but not as well as the never-married living with parents. Furstenberg and Crawford concluded, "Our analysis suggests that the assistance rendered by family members significantly alters the life chances of the young mother, enhancing her prospects of educational achievement and economic advancement."

In their review of research on the children of teenage parents Baldwin and Cain (1980) noted that a child's physical and cognitive development apparently could be improved by the presence of an adult in the household in addition to the young mother. Mednick (1979) reported that in a Danish population the physical status at one year of the babies of adolescent mothers who were raising the child alone was worse than that of those raised by a teenage mother and father, or a teenage mother and grandmother (mean scores of 9.2, 8.5, and 7.6—the higher the score the worse the health status). Furstenberg (1976) found that children of adolescent mothers scored higher on a Preschool Inventory if caretaking responsibility was shared with another adult, generally the child's grandmother, or another close relative. Kellam (1978, 1979) in a study of a low-income black community in Chicago indicated that the negative effects on school achievement of being born to an adolescent mother were ameliorated by the presence of either a father or a grandmother in the household. Baldwin and Cain concluded, "Research on the role of family structure strongly suggests that the presence of adults other than the young mother in some way mitigates the deleterious health and other effects on the child associated with teenage childbearing."

## SUPPORT FOR FAMILY CARE

The issue of adolescent childbearing needs to be examined from several perspectives. There seems little doubt that mother, father, child, family, and society would benefit from a delay in childbearing until young females and males have at least completed high school, received adequate vocational training, and married. Numerous studies make it abundantly clear that adolescent pregnancy is associated not only with increased maternal health risks, but also often leads to inadequate education, welfare dependency, and high completed fertility in the mother. It may also have adverse effects on the child and on its father. Thus society's first priority in this area should be prevention of early unplanned childbearing through whatever means possible, including family life education, contraception, and abortion.

Since it seems unlikely, however, that even widespread availability of such programs would completely eliminate adolescent childbearing, opportunities to minimize the consequences of such births must be considered. These should include the choice of living arrangements during pregnancy and in the years immediately following delivery. The evidence just presented suggests that most young mothers and their infants will benefit from living in a family with parents or other adult relatives. There will be situations, however, where family strife or individual psychopathology makes this impossible, therefore other facilities should be available including independent households, foster care, and group homes. Some young mothers may choose marriage and this choice must be allowed, although such marriages are very unstable, particularly when the male is also an adolescent. But, overall, social policy should favor family care.

Education and action are needed, however, if the percentage of adolescent mothers and children receiving family care is to be increased and if mothers, children, and families are to receive maximum support. Possible strategies include: (1) encouraging agencies serving pregnant adolescents and young parents to work with the adolescents' families; (2) providing counseling to families around the stresses of maintaining young mothers and their children in the household; (3) increasing the availability of day care services; and (4) insuring that welfare policies provide financial incentives for families that care for young mothers and their children.

## Agency Services

A large number of traditional agencies provide health, educational, welfare, social, and other services to pregnant adolescents and young mothers. In addition, in many large communities, comprehensive agencies have been developed recently whose exclusive focus is the provision or integration of multiple services to this population. This movement was encouraged by Public Law 95-626 passed in 1978 which provided grants for such programs. Forbush and Maciocha (1981), however, found that many of these programs did not actively incorporate family members in their service arrangements and they recommended greater involvement of families. The 1981 Adolescent Family Demonstration Projects addition to the Public Health Service Act (Title XX) places much more emphasis on involvement of the family. For example, all grant applications must include a description of how the applicant will "involve families of adolescents in a manner which will maximize the role of the family in the solution of problems relating to the parenthood or pregnancy of the adolescent."

Agencies that do not deal exclusively with pregnant adolescents and young mothers may be even less cognizant of the need to work with the entire family unit than are the specialized agencies. Federal and state governments, as well as voluntary organizations and professional associations, should increase their efforts to educate practitioners in many fields about the special needs of adolescent parents. In particular, they should attempt to increase workers' awareness of the potential positive influence of the adolescents' families and of what agencies can do to maximize this impact. (For additional suggestions in this area see the report of the Family Impact Seminar's study of teenage pregnancy, Ooms, 1981.)

## *Counseling*

Pregnant adolescents and their families need assistance not only in dealing with the trauma surrounding the pregnancy itself, but around the conflicts that can be expected to arise when a new mother-child unit is incorporated into a household. Counseling, sensitive to the special needs of this population, should be available during the prenatal period when decisions are being made and during the years of adjustment that follow. Individual casework may be appropriate in some cases, while family therapy may be needed in others. Adolescent concerns can sometimes be more easily expressed in group sessions with other pregnant females or young mothers. Nor should the needs of the young father and his family be ignored (Earls and Siegel, 1980; Parke et al., 1980).

New grandparents also may gain additional insights from participation in group sessions with others who are having similar experiences. For example, the Chicago Child Care Society has organized a Senior Parents' Group to assist black grandparents and older parents cope with child rearing (Stokes and Greenstone, 1981).

Discussing the role of the grandmother in adolescent pregnancy and parenting, Smith (1975) has commented:

By mobilizing support from significant figures in the young woman's own life and involving them in plans for her care and future support in rearing her family, we can ensure continuing fulfillment of her needs as she copes with the developmental tasks of motherhood. Often, especially for the adolescent mother, her own mother is the most significant figure. If a good relationship can be fostered between mother and daughter and the very normal conflicts between them eased, the young woman may be more able to complete her own education, fill her own developmental needs, and provide adequate mothering for her child. Understanding the concerns and problems of the mother of the pregnant adolescent and providing her with the supports that she needs in order to guide her daughter toward motherhood can often be the key to a healthy mother-child relationship between the adolescent mother and her infant. Simultaneously, the adolescent's mother may find gratification and pleasure in a new developmental phase in her life as she becomes a grandmother.

Furstenberg (1980a, 1980b, and 1981) also has noted that the birth of a grandchild and the needs of the young mother and her child may develop a new and stronger relationship between the daughter and her mother and siblings—and in fact strengthen the entire family unit, at least temporarily. The potential conflicts between this process and the normal adolescent striving for independence have yet to be studied.

Intensive counseling services are also essential to identify those situations in which it is in the best interests of the young mother and child to separate them from her family. Because of the shortage of trained caseworkers with adequate time to devote to these problems, many such decisions must be made on the basis of what the adolescent herself reports. Often she will recount real or anticipated scenes of conflict and even violence. If those responsible for advising the adolescent about living arrangements do not have the time to discuss the situation with the parents at the office or preferably at home, they will be forced to decide on the basis of inadequate information and short-range considerations, such as avoiding possible conflict. Only if sufficient resources are available to permit home visits, intensive counseling, group work, and other interventions is it possible to obtain the information necessary to balance short-term consequences against long-range benefits for the young mother, infant, and family—and, in the long run, society.

Some situations may require weekly or more frequent visits by a public health nurse or community outreach worker in addition to casework or therapy in order to protect the new mother and child and encourage the development of relationships which will promote the physical and emotional growth of the new mother and child. The advantages of such interventions probably will outweigh their costs. (For an example of a successful program, see Field et al., 1980.)

## Day Care

In households where the grandmother works, infant and preschool day care may be the only solution to the problem of how the new mother is to complete her education and/or job training. Even if the grandmother is not employed, day care may be needed on a respite basis if she is not to feel overburdened, with deleterious effects on both the infant and its mother.

Unfortunately, day care is in short supply in many areas, and particularly day care for infants. A recent survey of services provided by agencies serving pregnant and parenting adolescents revealed that day care was one of the services least often provided (JRB Associates, 1981), although many other studies have indicated that both agencies and young mothers afford it high priority (American Institute for Research, 1979; Goldstein and Wallace, 1978).

Moreover, many day care facilities are not adapted to the particular needs of the adolescent mother who is attending school. For example, to serve a student-mother such facilities must open very early and be available by public transportation. Day care providers need to realize the inexperience of the young mother and be prepared to spend more time explaining observed problems than they would with older or more experienced mothers. The grandmother also may have to be involved when special needs are revealed.

Agencies planning the allocation of day care services should be aware of the numbers of adolescent mothers and children in their communities. Their need for day care services may be as acute as the need among older mothers, yet they may be less able to make their problems known to decision-makers.

## Income Support

Despite variations in welfare policies from state to state and differences in interpretation within states, the general thrust of state AFDC and Medicaid policies is to encourage pregnant adolescents and young mothers to remain in their parents' households. (Moore, 1979). The financial incentive is not large, however, and occasionally is absent or negative (Cartoof, 1982; Furstenberg, 1980b).

Federal and state governments, therefore, should review welfare policies and their implementation to make certain that they encourage families to care for the new mother-infant unit. There should be recognition of the fact that the addition of a grandchild may bring more economic and other strains than if the grandmother herself had another child. For example, the grandmother's childbearing cycle already may have been concluded and therefore all infant supplies (furniture, clothes, etc.) may have been given away. In addition, the grandmother may now be employed. Also, the new mother is no longer only a child. Her needs for physical space for herself and her infant must be considered. Overcoming such problems requires additional economic support, and determination on the part of welfare workers to attempt to solve emotional and other difficulties rather than establishing a separate household.

## CONCLUSIONS

The number of adolescents bearing children probably will decrease in the next few decades as the number of adolescents declines and the use of contraceptives and abortions becomes more widespread unless access to these two services is restricted, as is currently being proposed. Adolescent parenting, however, will remain a significant social welfare problem and one contributing to the number of three generation households.

During the 1960s and 1970s, comprehensive service programs were developed to meet some of the needs of the young mother and her child. Initially focused on the prenatal and immediate postpartum period, these programs were concerned primarily with the health of mother and infant and the mother's education and welfare status. Increasingly, social policy is examining the wider consequences of the problem in terms of the social and emotional development of mother and child, and the impact of the new unit on the child's father, on families, and on society across a longer time span.

Within these frameworks the influence and importance of the family has gained new prominence. Public Law 95-626, which established the grant program for supporting adolescent pregnancy projects, lists "counseling for extended family members of the eligible person" as a suggested supplemental service and gives priority to applicants who involve the community to be served, including adolescents and families, in the planning and implementation of the projects. The new Adolescent Family Demonstration Projects Act places even greater emphasis on family involvement. The Family Impact Seminar, a program of the George Washington University's Institute for Educational Leadership, has examined the issues surrounding teenage pregnancy and developed recommendations about needed research and policy implementation from a family perspective (Ooms, 1981). The Administration for Children, Youth, and Families, the Center for Population Research of the National Institute for Child Health and Human Development, and the Office of Adolescent Pregnancy Programs (all within the federal Department of Health and Human Services) are focusing increased attention on the family of the pregnant adolescent and the young mother as an underutilized resource in coping with the problems of adolescent parenting.

Long-term analyses suggest that funds allocated to helping families maintain young mothers and their infants within their households will have financial and other benefits. Welfare costs should be lower when one rather than two households are supported. Completion of high school education and job training is more likely for the adolescent mother, and sometimes even the adolescent father, when they remain in a family setting, thus increasing the possibility of their employment and welfare independence. Living with their families often delays additional childbearing among young mothers in comparison to those who live independently or with a male partner. In addition, physical and cognitive development in infants appears to be enhanced by the three generation household.

Continuing advocacy at federal, state, and local levels is essential to convert public and professional concern and research findings into social policies and programs.

## REFERENCES

American Institutes for Research. *The Ecology of Help-Seeking Behavior Among Adolescent Parents*. Cambridge, 1979.

Baldwin, W. and Cain, V.S. The Chidlren of Teenage Parents. *Family Planning Perspectives*, 12:34-43, 1980.

Cartoof, V. The Negative Effects of AFDC Policies on Teenage Mothers. *Child Welfare*. 61:269-278, 1982.

Centers for Disease Control. Childbearing and Abortion Patterns Among Teenagers—United States, 1978. *Morbidity and Mortality Weekly Report*, 30:616-620, 1981.

Coleman, J.S. Preface. *Youth: Transition to Adulthood*. (Report of the Panel on Youth of the President's Science Advisory Committee.) Chicago: The University of Chicago Press, 1974.

Earls, F. and Siegel, B. Precocious Fathers. *American Journal of Orthopsychiatry*, 50: 469-480, 1980.

Ezzard, N.V. et al. Race-Specific Patterns of Abortion Use by American Teenagers. *American Journal of Public Health*. 72:809-814, 1982.

Field, T.M. et al. Teenage, Lower-Class, Black Mothers and Their Preterm Infants: An Intervention and Developmental Follow-Up. *Child Development*. 51:426-436, 1980.

Forbush, J.B. and Maciocha, T. Adolescent Parent Programs and Family Involvement. In Ooms, T. (ed.), *Teenage Pregnancy in a Family Context: Implications for Policy*. Philadelphia: Temple University Press, 1981.

Furstenberg, F.F., Jr. and Crawford, A.C. Family Support: Helping Teenage Mothers to Cope. *Family Planning Perspectives*, 10:322-333, 1978.

Furstenberg, F.F., Jr. *Unplanned Parenthood: The Social Consequences of Teenage Childbearing*. New York: Free Press, 1976.

Furstenberg, F.F., Jr. *Teenage Parenthood and Family Support*. Paper prepared for the National Research Forum on Family Issues sponsored by the White House Conference on Families, Washington D.C., April 10-11, 1980(a).

Furstenberg, F.F., Jr. Burdens and Benefits: The Impact of Early Childbearing on the Family. *Journal of Social Issues*. 36:64-87, 1980(b).

Furstenberg, F.F., Jr. Implicating the Family: Teenage Parenthood and Kinship Involvement. In Ooms, T. (ed.), *Teenage Pregnancy in a Family Context: Implications for Policy*. Philadelphia: Temple University Press, 1981.

Goldstein, H. and Wallace, H.M. Services and Needs of Pregnant Teenagers in Large Cities of the United States, 1976. *Public Health Reports*, 93:46-54, 1978.

Gorbach, J. and Messenger, K. Personal communication.

JRB Associates: *Final Report on National Study of Teenage Pregnancy*. McLean, VA 1981.

Kellam, S.G. *Consequences of Teenage Motherhood for Mother, Child, and Family in a Black Urban Community*. Progress Reports to National Institute of Child Health and Human Development, July 1978 and June 1979.

Kinard, E.M. and Klerman, L.V. Teenage Parenting and Child Abuse: Are They Related? *American Journal of Orthopsychiatry*, 50:481-488, 1980.

Leishman, K. Teenage Mothers Are Keeping Their Babies—With the Help of Their Own Mothers. *MS*, 61-67, 1980.

Leventhal, J.M. Risk Factors for Child Abuse: Methodologic Standards in Case-Control Studies. *Pediatrics*, 68:684-690, 1981.

Mednick, B.R. *Consequences of Family Structure and Maternal State for Child and Mother's Development*. Progress Reports to National Institute of Child Health and Human Development, January and July 1979.

Moore, K.A. *Policy Determinants of Teenage Childbearing*. Progress Report to National Institute of Child Health and Human Development, 1979.

*Newsweek*. The Baby Boomers Come of Age. Pages 34-37, March 30, 1981.

O'Connell, M. and Moore, M.J. The Legitimacy of First Births to U.S. Women Aged 15-24, 1939-1978. *Family Planning Perspectives*, 12:16-25, 1980.

Ooms, T. (ed.) *Teenage Pregnancy in a Family Context: Implications for Policy*. Philadelphia: Temple University Press, 1981.

Parke, R.D. et al. The Adolescent Father's Impact on the Mother and Child. *Journal of Social Issues*, 36:88-106, 1980.

Public Health Service: *Health, United States, 1981*. Hyattsville, MD: U.S. Department of Health and Human Services, 1981. (DHHS Publication No. (PHS) 82-1232.)

Rauh, J.H. et al. The Reproductive Adolescent. *Pediatric Clinics of North America*, 20: 1005-1020, 1973.

Smith, D.S. Life Course, Norms, and the Family System of Older Americans in 1900. *Journal of Family History*, 4:285-298, 1979.

Smith, E.W. The Role of the Grandmother in Adolescent Pregnancy and Parenting. *Journal of School Health*, 45:278-282, 1975.

Stokes, J. and Greenstone J. Helping Black Grandparents and Older Parents Cope with Child Rearing: A Group Method. *Child Welare*, 60:691-701, 1981.

Trudeau, G.B. Doonesbury strip published in *Boston Sunday Globe*, May 4, 1980.

Wallace, H.M. et al. The Maternity Home: Present Services and Future Roles. *American Journal of Public Health*, 64:568-575, 1974.

Zelnik, M. and Kantner, J.F. First Pregnancies to Women Age 15-19: 1976 and 1971. *Family Planning Perspectives*, 10:11-20, 1978.

Zelnik, M. and Kantner, J.F. Sexual Activity, Contraceptive Use and Pregnancy Among Metropolitan-Area Teenagers: 1971-1979. *Family Planning Perspectives*, 12:230-237, 1980.

# Who Should Control
# Long-Term Planning
# for the Elderly?

Alan Sager

## *INTRODUCTION*

When an older person becomes frail, disabled, or confused, long-term care is often needed. Decisions must then be made about the goals of long-term care, the site(s) in which it should be provided, and the types, quantities, and providers of services needed to reach goals chosen at the site(s) selected.

These decisions can be difficult to make well. There are several explanations for this state of affairs. First, the goals of long-term care can be difficult to articulate, for both practical and emotional reasons. Second, once articulated, goals may be difficult to agree about. Third, even after reaching agreement on goals, uncertainty remains about the costs and benefits of long-term care in different settings, employing services of varying types and intensity. This uncertainty is attributable largely to the practical and ethical problems of conducting research into the efficacy of long-term care or learning what services are needed by which patients.

Under those circumstances, there is room for both speculation and collection of evidence regarding appropriate roles for patients, families, and different professionals in deciding the goals, settings, and proper services for long-term care. Following a brief discussion of obstacles to knowledge-building in long-term care, this chapter will consider the claims which can be advanced for and against

This chapter is based in part on studies funded by the U.S. Adminstration on Aging, Office of Human Development Services, Department of Health, Education, and Welfare (grants 90-1026-01-02) and by the National Retired Teachers Association–American Association of Retired Persons' Andrus Foundation. It does not necessarily reflect the views of either organization. The comments of Thomas R. Willemain, James J. Callahan, Jr., and Robert Perlman on earlier versions of this chapter are greatly appreciated.

*129*

assigning influence to each of the three parties. It will present new data on the merits of these claims, and then suggest an approach to cooperative long-term planning.

*Obstacles to knowledge-building.* There appear to be four principal obstacles to knowledge-building in long-term care: difficulties in measuring outcomes; ethical and practical problems in applying experimental techniques; non-comparability of individual research findings; and the inter-dependence between who is permitted influence over long-term care (goals, sites, and services) and the outcomes or effectiveness of care itself.

The condition of an older person needing long-term care can be difficult to measure objectively. Unless status in important dimensions can be reliably and validly described, attribution of change in status to service is impossible. Natural changes in condition usually evolve slowly; services are seldom expected to result in cure; and the impacts of services are often difficult to measure. The last is particularly true when services are designed to slow the declines in functioning that accompany deterioration of such chronic medical problems as arthritis. Conventional outcome measures in acute medicine—saving a life or controlling an illness—are often not useful in long-term care. Similarly, changes in functional ability (independence in ordinary activities of daily living) do not reflect the effectiveness of most long-term care. Rather, 80-90 percent of care is designed to substitute for deficits in functional ability: helping a frail person walk or eat, for example. We are only beginning to develop reliable techniques for measuring the effectiveness of such services, and for linking their success to preventing, repairing, or slowing deterioration in medical, functional, and emotional well-being.

Were good outcome measures available, it would still be hard to learn what services, in what settings, were effective. Prospective experiments are difficult to construct because of the large sample sizes required to control for a large number of variables and for ongoing changes in status, and because patients should be followed for a considerable time in order to observe the often-subtle changes in well-being associated with long-term care services. Further, on both ethical and practical grounds, it is hard to seek or obtain informed consent for experimental manipulation of long-term care services for the elderly.

Retrospective matching may be a useful alternative to the prospective controlled experiment. Unless similar patients can be found in different settings, this method is more useful in comparing effectiveness of services in a given setting, such as the nursing home or the home itself. Here too, large samples are necessary to control simultaneously for the many medical, functional, emotional, economic, and programmatic variables which cannot be manipulated.

If past long-term care demonstration and research efforts had employed common patient and service variables, measured in similar ways, the data collected through these projects could have been summed to yield pictures of which services work under which circumstances. Future demonstrations should employ common assessment instruments to record objective patient characteristics, common definitions and techniques for measuring services, and common devices for recording changes in well-being over time.

A final obstacle to knowledge-building has to do with two distinct sorts of interactions. First, comparative cost and effectiveness of home and nursing home care, for example, probably depend in large measure on the goals sought and services provided in either setting. Second, there is probably a relation between who is permitted to influence goal, setting, and services and the outcome of care. These interactions figure prominently among the claims of various parties to influence over long-term care planning.

## *WHAT ARE THE CLAIMS OF PATIENTS, FAMILIES, AND PROFESSIONALS?*

In view of these obstacles, it is not surprising that we lack strong evidence on the comparative cost of home and nursing home care, or on the types and intensity of care required by different people in either setting.* Absent solid evidence on cost or effectiveness of

---

*See, for example Alan Sager, *Planning Home Care with the Elderly*, Cambridge: Ballinger, forthcoming 1982, and "Critical Review of Research on Long-term Care Alternatives Sponsored by the Department of Health, Education, and Welfare," Washington: Office of Assistant Secretary for Planning and Evaluation, DHEW, June 1977; New York State Moreland Act Commission, *Reimbursing Operating Costs* and *Assessment and Placement: Anything Goes*, Reports 5 and 6, New York: The Commission, March 1976; and Peter Kihss, "Point System of Reclassifying Nursing-Home Patients is Under Attack," *New York Times*, December 20, 1977.

Reviews of cost issues are found in Nancy Robinson, Eugene Shinn, Esther Adam, and Florence Moore, "Costs of Homemaker-Home Health Aide and Alternative Forms of Service: A Survey of the Literature," New York: National Council for Homemaker-Home Health Aide Services, Inc., 1974; "Cost Analysis: Home Health Care as an Alternative to Institutional Care," Kalamazoo, Michigan: Homemakers Upjohn, October 1975; General Accounting Office, letter to Rep. Edward I. Koch, MWO-76-30, B-164031(3), 17 September

home and nursing home care, or on needed services, the claims to influence over long-term care planning by patients, families, and various professionals should be examined.

The following discussion characterizes the arguments for and against influence by various groups as a "debate." While such a debate is seldom articulated, it is implicit in many long-term care proposals. To suggest use of vouchers is to assume that it is sensible to permit considerable patient influence. On the other hand, to focus on improved assessment forms and case management procedures is to place predominant trust in professionals.

First to be considered is influence over goals. Different individuals are likely to select as outcomes for long-term care enhanced longevity, improved functional ability, maintenance in comfort, safety, and others. No one outcome will usually be sought to the exclusion of others; rather, some mixture will be preferred. Patients, families, and professionals are likely to differ on the weights assigned to various goals for individual patients. They may differ systematically as well. Any party not content with the mixture of outcomes to be sought may be expected to actively rebel against the plan of care, or to passively withhold cooperation in implementing it.

Depending on the goal(s) sought, different treatment plans will be constructed. These will vary in their mixture of medical, therapeutic, nursing, and less skilled services. Different plans will be more or less costly, and comparative costs are likely to vary by setting. Plans to reach some goals (such as longevity and safety) for some patients might be less expensive to fulfill at home. Thus, an interaction among who is permitted to select goals, who designs service plans, cost of care, and lower-cost setting can be expected to occur.

Given widespread public dissatisfaction with the pronounced institutional emphasis in long-term care benefits for the elderly in the United States, combined with equally widespread official fears that more generous entitlement to non-institutional services will quickly prove insupportably expensive, one suggested approach has been to pay for expanded home care benefits only on behalf of those who would otherwise require nursing home care which was

---

1975; and John Craig, "Cost Issues in Home Health Care," in Marie Callender and Judy LaVor, *Home Health Development, Problems and Potential*, Washington: Disability and Long-term Care Study, Office of the Assistant Secretary for Planniing and Evaluation, Department of Health, Education and Welfare, April 1975, pp. 48-55.

at least as expensive. Given the issues discussed above, whose views of needed in-home services (and their cost) should be expressed for purposes of comparison?

Even when a goal or constellation of goals is agreed to, if patients, family members, and different professionals differ in their judgment of services needed to reach that goal, whose views should prevail? Costs of the plans can be estimated, but what about their likely effectiveness? Speculations on the likely cost and effectiveness of plans designed by members of each group now follow. Subsequently, data from a recent study bearing on these speculations are reported, and the advantages and disadvantages of assigning influence to the different parties are discussed.

It might be claimed on *patient's* behalf that most long-term care services, which substitute for functional deficits, simply constitute replacements for things patients have done for themselves since childhood. Patients can therefore be expected to have good ideas of what they need help with and how much help they need. These ordinary activities—assistance with mobility, cleaning, bathing, cooking, and the like—are not technical; they are the kinds of services about which we permit people as consumers to exercise sovereignty in spending their own money.

Further, at a time when patients' economic resources and physical and cognitive strength are sometimes diminishing, weakening of influence or deprivation of control over management of these ordinary activities can be particularly frustrating. Control by others can reduce self-esteem and increase feelings of helplessness, depression, or rage. The alternative, allowing patient influence over home care planning, should help patients become or remain active participants in their own care, rather than passive recipients of services. The in-home services might themselves be more effective, and there may be spillover benefits, as patients feel and act more autonomously in other spheres.

This may apply particularly to patients' loss of control over the setting of care—over housing arrangements. Many older people resent having to move in with children or siblings as the price for obtaining safe, regular care from relatives, and thereby avoiding institutionalization. For a patient lacking family who are able and willing to provide care, or whose family requires the support of paid in-home services, the right to influence the types, quantities, and providers of those paid in-home services could be an important means of holding home care's cost below that of the institution. This influence could involve deciding a) what help is needed (cooking, bathing, transferring, and so on), b) how much help with each service is called for weekly or monthly, and/or c) which providers, with what skills, are required to give various types of assistance.

Against patient influence or control over home care planning, parallel arguments can be advanced: patients do not know or cannot be trusted to say what they need; it is unfair to permit patients the "autonomy" that could oblige them to design home care plans whose costs fall below those of the nursing home.

On the question of knowledge, critics of patient influence assert that while many patients may know what level of well-being they would like to enjoy, they cannot be expected to decide how much help, from which providers, is required to reach that level. Further, how is it to be decided which patients' preferences are to be respected? Some may well be confused. If an individual patient is deemed generally competent, should s/he have the right to select services which do not appear important to professionals?

Regarding trust, it may be feared that some patients are overdemanding; they will seek more service than is really needed. Much home care consists of help provided in past centuries to the wealthy by servants. Assistance in cleaning the house or in shopping may be desired by some who do not need it, when a public program pays the bill. (Indeed, the institutional emphasis in public long-term care, generally disliked by the elderly, can be seen as a device to control utilization.)

Against this fear of overuse of services by some, it may be suspected than other older people cannot be trusted to plan care because they will deny needs for help (because they do not wish to admit dependence, do not wish to be a burden on others, or simply do not want strangers in their home), and are therefore, likely to request dangerously low levels of service.

If expanded home care benefits are to be available to prospective nursing home entrants only when those benefits will cost less than institutional care to be provided, it may not be appropriate, in many cases, to ask frail, ill, and frightened older people to choose their home care service plans. It may be hard to decide when patients are safely able to plan care on their own behalf. A scheme for patient autonomy in long-term care planning may become in some circumstances a means by which patients are induced to accept less help than they believe they really need, as the price of avoiding entry to the nursing home.

Finally, some patients may be reassured by being told by an authoritative professional (wearing a white coat or other uniform) just what services are needed to make her or him well. Deprived of this placebo effect through forced involvement in planning their own care, they may be less likely to recover from an illness or enjoy peace-of-mind. This points to the need to identify patients for whom influence over home care planning is appropriate.

Many of the arguments for and against patient involvement apply to the *family* as well. Therefore, only those aspects of participation which pertain particularly to the family are now noted. There is one powerful reason to support family claims for influence in long-term care planning, one reason to oppose it, and one area of potentially frequent and deep family-patient conflict to be discussed.

Family participation in long-term care planning should improve the likelihood that arrangements and services decided on will be acceptable to the family. Family's satisfaction with the level of formal support is likely to be central to their own continued will-ingness to care. Too much paid help may threaten a family's perceived responsibility for its older member and may be seen as an unwelcome intrusion into the home, while too little paid help may challenge the family to do more than it is really able, resulting either in frantic efforts to do "enough" for the patient or in inade-quate care, or in a family's decision to institutionalize the older person.

Some administrators and legislators fear that family influence in long-term care planning is likely to result in widespread lobbying for "inappropriately" high levels of paid services, and consequent abandonment or shedding of many families' caring functions. Given the large share of long-term care now provided by families at home, even small reductions in family effort are likely to yield large proportionate increases in the need for paid long-term care services. It may be that the perceived horror or shame of the nurs-ing home admission has helped spur high levels of family home care. To allow family influence in planning formal home care ser-vices could therefore open an avenue by which families could in good conscience withdraw some significant share of their support of older patients.

It is easy to describe one goal of paid in-home services: to support patients' self-care and families' informal support, not to weaken them or to substitute for them inappropriately. It is hard, however, to discover if (and, if so, what level of) family participation in planning paid services is likely to promote attainment of this goal.

Because the "debate" over who should control the planning of long-term care is sometimes posed as fundamentally a competition between consumers (patients and families) and providers (various professionals), it can be easy to overlook the opportunities for disagreement between a patient and her/his family. The most profound disagreement is usually over site of care, and over the amount of paid in-home help needed to forestall nursing home admission. A family which has tired of the burden of home care may demand high levels of paid in-home support as the price for continuing to keep an aged parent at home. This is particularly likely when the parent is incontinent, confused, and/or on bad terms with the family. The patient may feel that little paid help is needed, or may simply prefer to be cared for by the family members. More starkly, the family may refuse to keep the patient at home any longer, and the patient may refuse to enter a nursing home. The conflicting human and legal rights of the two parties, and the practical difficulties of enforcing either right, often preclude solutions satisfactory to both parties.

Advocates of *professional* influence over long-term care planning can marshall impressive arguments, but must contend with important criticisms as well. The complexity of long-term care, experience and knowledge about what works, and the desire for equity all support professionals' claims to influence. While many forms of long-term care are mundane substitutes for deficits in patients' own functional ability, the organization of these substitutes and their coordination with skilled care by physicians, nurses, PTs, OTs, social workers, dieticians, and others can be complex tasks. Even if coordination is not called for, patients and families may know that help is needed in a given mundane area, such as meal preparation, but they may not know the most efficient or effective means of preparation.

Further, professionals, having observed the impact of various types, quantities, and providers of long-term care on patients and families in different circumstances, may be expected to know what forms of help are likely to be effective in a given case.

Finally, professional influence is likely to be the best vehicle for assuring both horizontal and vertical equity—that patients with similar needs are treated similarly, and that patients who need more help get more help.

Contending against professionals' claims are arguments that it is too expensive and time-consuming to assemble all the pertinent experts to design a patient's long-term care plan, that professional influence is likely to undermine patients' and families' own needs for some measure of autonomy, and that inconsistency or unreliability of professional judgment in other fields (where agreement should be easier to achieve than in long-term care) suggests that professionals may not find it easy to design effective or equitable home care plans. The last argument merits elaboration.

Consistency of professional judgment does not ensure validity or accuracy (judges may be grouped in a tight pattern two yards from the true bull's-eye). But if professional judgments are widely scattered, the chance that any one expert's home care plan is on target seems remote. Given the difficulties of measuring outcomes or of learning what services are effective, how is it to be decided which of varied professional views are likely to be correct? Professional reliability would at least point to a possible location of the true target—the "right" package of services—whose effectiveness could then be tested experimentally. The following section reports the results of a study designed both to seek this target and to collect indirect evidence on the likely costs and effectiveness of home care plans designed by patients, their families, and various professionals.*

## ASSESSING THE MERITS OF PATIENT, FAMILY, AND PROFESSIONAL INFLUENCE

Fifty patients about to be discharged from six Massachusetts hospitals to nursing homes were studied. Patients and family members were separately interviewed. They were asked which of 41 services would be required to sustain the patient at home in a "safe, adequate, and dignified manner," how often the services would be needed, and whether unpaid providers could deliver the help. Because patients had lived at home prior to this hospital admission, it was felt that they and their families would have available the basis for a realistic judgment of home care needs.

Professional views of service requirements were sought as well. To test professional consistency, the detailed, independent judg-

---

*Alan Sager, *Planning Home Care with the Elderly,* Cambridge: Ballinger, forthcoming, 1982.

ments of eighteen different care planners were obtained. A modified version of the "Patient Appraisal and Care Evaluation" (PACE) form was completed for each patient shortly before hospital discharge.* Functional, psychosocial, and medical characteristics of patients were recorded. Nine professionals—three physicians, three hospital discharge planners, and three home care agency planners—relied exclusively on the PACE to design hypothetical home care plans. Six additional professionals received the PACE, and also made brief visits to about half of the patients. These fifteen consultant professionals wrote care plans for each patient. Three additional in-hospital professionals—the patient's own physician, discharge planner, and primary nurse—received the PACE and relied also on their own detailed knowledge of the patient in designing care plans. For 20 of the 50 patients, interviews were completed with both patients and family members. The following sections comparing likely costs and effectiveness of patient, family, and professional views concern these 20 patients, unless otherwise noted.

*Comparing costs.* Home care costs depend on the volume of paid help provided. Patients, families, and professionals were asked to indicate the number of episodes of help in each of 41 services, and the shares of these which unpaid and paid providers could deliver. (An "episode" is a unit of service, such as giving a bath, cooking a meal, or monitoring vital signs.)

As Table 1 indicates, patients, family members, and professionals requested similar total numbers of episodes of help weekly, but they differed markedly in their requests for paid help. Professionals felt that considerably more paid help was necessary than did the others.

Interestingly, family members' estimates of their own (unpaid) contributions were the highest, both absolutely and proportionately. Neither families' nor patients' service requests fit the "demanding consumer" model.

Across the full study sample of 50 patients, about half could have been diverted from nursing home to home care with no increase in total cost, based on professionals' views of needed services. While the costs of services sought by patients and family members could not be precisely compared with the cost of institu-

---

*Ellen W. Jones, Barbara J. McNitt, and Eleanor M. McKnight, *Patient Classification for Long-term Care: User's Manual,* Department of HEW Publication No. HRA 74-3107, Washington: Bureau of Health Services Research and Evaluation, December, 1973.

Table 1

Patient, Family, and Professional Views of
Home Care Needs

| Need As Viewed By | Weekly Episodes of Help (mean) | | |
|---|---|---|---|
| | Total | Paid | % Paid |
| Patients | 118 | 75 | 63.6% |
| Families | 130 | 72 | 55.4% |
| Professionals | 130 | 92 | 70.8% |

n = 20

tional care,* non-professionals' relatively modest requests for paid
services suggest that home care would be even more competitive,
were their views respected. If patients and their families were in
practice allowed to choose home care only when it cost no more
than the institutional alternative, greater patient/family influence
over home care planning would probably permit more to choose
home care itself. Because these findings are based on small samples
of patients, families, and professionals, and because the home care
planning is itself hypothetical, additional evidence would be most
helpful.

To try to learn if the less-expensive, non-professional home care
plans were bought at the price of reduced effectiveness, this study
sought to gauge the possible outcomes of patients', families', and
professionals' home care plans.

*Comparing effectiveness.* Three procedures were used to try to
measure the likely outcome or effectiveness of patient, family, and

*This was because less detailed information was sought from patients and family members (in the interest of human subjects' protection).

professional home care plans. First, allocation of requested help among different types of service was examined, on the assumption that outcomes would depend partly on the types of service sought. Second, the relation of requested help to patient functional ability was analyzed to learn if help was prescribed in an apparently reasonable relation to need. Third, the reliability of professionals themselves was examined in several ways, because it was believed that greater consistency would point to greater validity of prescribed care. The first two of these approaches are now pursued; the third is taken up in the next section.

As Table 1 indicated, the three groups of care planners differed but little in their views of total service need. Similarly, it was found that the proportions of total episodes of help thought necessary by each of the care planners across four major service groupings were strikingly similar (see Table 2). The same was found for distributions of paid help. This indicates that the three groups agreed well about needed services; the major area of disagreement concerned the number of episodes of unpaid versus paid personal care thought necessary. Agreement about episodes of nursing and medical-therapeutic services was striking, as Table 2 indicates.

The second method of estimating likely effectiveness of patient, family, and professional care plans was to measure the relation between each group's requested episodes and patients' functional ability at discharge. It was hypothesized that effective care plans would typically show an inverse relation between the volume of prescribed services and functional ability: this would acknowledge that more disabled people typically needed more help, and that less disabled people could be made inappropriately dependent if they received too much help. Functional ability was measured by the Barthel score, a zero-to-one hundred scale of independence in ordinary activities of daily living.

Patients, their families, and professionals all sought home care whose intensity varied inversely with patient functional ability. The Pearson product-moment correlations for the three groups were $-0.62$, $-0.57$, and $-0.76$, respectively. All relations would have been expected by chance fewer than once in one hundred times (one-tail test).

In summary, this study's findings suggest that, in the area of cost, patients and family members appear unlikely to design unreasonable home care plans. Their requests would probably cost less than those of professionals. The expectations of family members

Table 2

Total and Paid Episodes Distributed
Among Major Service Types

### A. Weekly Episodes of Help, Total

| Need As Viewed By | Personal Care | House-Keeping | Nursing | Medical-Therapeutic | TOTAL |
|---|---|---|---|---|---|
| Patients | 60 | 32 | 23 | 3 | 118 |
| Families | 70 | 29 | 27 | 4 | 130 |
| Professionals | 71 | 34 | 22 | 3 | 130 |

### B. Paid Weekly Episodes of Help

| | | | | | |
|---|---|---|---|---|---|
| Patients | 43 | 16 | 13 | 3 | 75 |
| Families | 36 | 15 | 17 | 4 | 72 |
| Professionals | 52 | 20 | 17 | 3 | 92 |

n = 20

regarding maintenance of unpaid help at high levels are especially important in this regard: While patients' requests would have cost less than professionals' to fulfill, because the former simply sought less help, families' requests were cheaper than professionals' only because families expected that a high proportion of help would be provided by unpaid helpers.

In the area of suggested effectiveness of home care plans as well, this study's results are fairly encouraging to advocates of selective consumer influence over long-term care planning. The three groups differed but little in their average estimates of needed weekly episodes of care—both in total and in four major service groupings. Further, all three sets of care planners sought help in inverse relation to patient functional ability. This indicates that, on average, all groups conceived of home care needs in an apparently reasonable manner.

While the true effectiveness of these hypothetical home care plans cannot be gauged, the similarities between patient and family views, on average, and the relatively high Pearson correlation between them of 0.67, in individual cases, suggest that relatively little conflict between patient and family might be expected. One area of conflict might concern the specific jobs which paid providers might be asked to do, such as bathing or dressing. Family members may be reluctant to do unpleasant jobs or difficult jobs, such as bathing, but patients may be least willing to accept aid from strangers with these sorts of services.

Between patient/family views, and those of professionals, average agreement about needs in the four major service groupings was good. On average, then, to allow influence to patients and families would not seem to yield total levels of help or gross distributions of help by service groupings markedly different from those prescribed by professionals. Differences in individual cases are attributable largely to varying allocation of total hours of help between paid and unpaid services.

If relatively small differences can be expected in the cost and effectiveness of patients', families', and professionals' home care plans, closer looks at the reliability and validity of professionals' views are called for. This serves two purposes. First, since patients, families, and professionals happen to agree about home care service needs fairly well, it is useful to know if they are all right or all wrong. Second, if professionals are themselves inconsistent in their home care planning, this unreliability would undermine the presumed effectiveness of the typical professional's home care plan. The door would then be opened to a greater measure of patient/family influence over home care planning, at no apparent increase in cost and relatively little risk of reduced effectiveness.

*Assessing professionals' reliability and validity.* If professionals agree well about the home care needs of the elderly, this would point to the possibility that prescribed services would be effective. And, given the difficulty of directly measuring effectiveness of long-term care services, this pointer would be most welcome. If professionals do not generally agree, it would be desirable to explore when they do agree and, if possible, why. This would indicate opportunities for improving reliability in the future. Multiple clusters of views, if they were found to exist, would suggest opportunities for clinical trials or natural experiments to learn which group is right.

There are four potential sources of disagreement among professionals about the hypothetical home care needs of the elderly patients who comprise the sample of the study described above.

First, the phrase "safe, adequate, and dignified" may be interpreted to mean service at different levels in different areas of home care. Goals may vary; household services may matter more to one professional; continuous supervision and medical monitoring may matter more to another.

Second, given agreement about goals, professionals may synthesize the discrete objective data about patients into varying pictures of overall condition and need.

Third, given agreement about goals and current status, professionals may disagree about prognosis, the path the patient might take absent care.

Finally, even given agreement about the foregoing, professionals could still disagree about the types, quantities, and providers of home care required to move the patient from current status along a desired trajectory toward particular goals. In view of these opportunities for disagreement, it is not surprising that a considerable mixture of consistency and variation was found in professional prescriptions.

There really is no *a priori* way to identify when agreement fades to disagreement. Rather, it must be decided in specific instances whether the extent of agreement which may be expected is sufficient for the purpose at hand. Even weak agreement suffices to support parimutuel wagering on horse races; somewhat better agreement on rules of ordinary behavior is adequate to govern Boston-area auto drivers (except at rotaries); but only excellent agreement among engineers will persuade public authority bond underwriters that a bridge will support investors' financial risks.

Professional agreement was best at more aggregated levels and declined steadily as service plans were examined more discretely. The groups of professionals—physicians, nurses, and social workers—agreed very well about the needs of the average patient overall. They agreed less well about average need for help with specific services, such as bathing or physical therapy. The professional groups' consistency about individual patients' needs for specific services was worse still. Finally, agreement among the consultants about individual patients' requirements for help with specific services was apparently worst of all. These data indicate inconsistency among professional views of home care need.

Factor analysis was performed to learn if patterns of agreement among professionals could be identified. Only weak clustering by training was found. Role (discharge planning or home care planning) was not a unifying element. Generally, agreement across lines of professional training was stronger than it was within a profession. Certain doctors, nurses, and social workers formed clusters of shared views of needed home care.

Kendall's W and Cronbach's alpha tests were also used to measure agreement. These revealed surprising patterns of consistency beneath the apparent disagreement. Some professionals prescribed relatively high numbers of hours across patients; others, relatively few hours. Professionals were able to agree well about *which* patients needed more help or less help—their disagreement concerned *how much* help a given patient required. Each professional had his/her own yardstick, but applied it in a similar manner. Figure 1 illustrates this notion by presenting the five physicians' views of five typical patients.

Another support for some measure of professional influence over home care planning can be found in the results of regression analyses. The mean number of hours prescribed by professionals for a given patient was the dependent variable, and patient characteristics were the independent variables. Three patient characteristics—functional ability, age, and psychosocial well-being—"explained" over three-fourths of the difference in prescribed hours across patients ($R^2 = .754$; significant at less than .001). This indicates that the average of professionally prescribed hours bore a very reasonable and consistent relation to patient characteristics.

This evidence of prescribing home care in a consistent relation to patient characteristics, and the good agreement among professionals about patients' relative needs for care together indicate an underlying reasonableness of professional decision-making. What remains lacking however, is consensus about either the overall need for help by a specific patient, or about the services required.

## SUMMARY AND CONCLUSIONS

What are the meanings of the above findings for the partitioning of influence or control over home care planning? All three groups—

FIGURE 1

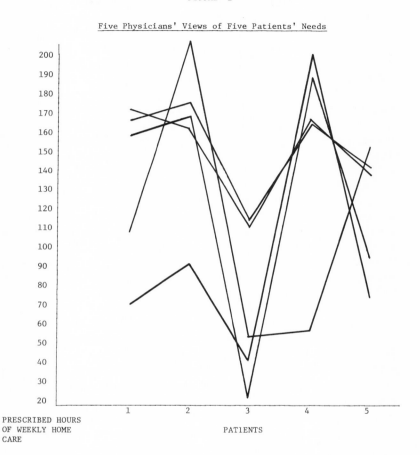

Five Physicians' Views of Five Patients' Needs

PRESCRIBED HOURS
OF WEEKLY HOME              PATIENTS
CARE

patients, families, and professionals—seem to recommend care in reasonable and equitable ways. Professional reliability, particularly about total need for care, seems good in many respects. But, as we expected following a general review of reliability in several fields, professional consistency in home care is not unbroken. Indeed, considering the general obstacles to consistency and the special attributes of long-term care which had been expected to further weaken interprofessional agreement, care planners seem to have acted with surprising congruence.

Partisans of consumers (patients and family) or professionals may seize on selected analyses to support their positions, but no

dramatic evidence really has been uncovered for or against dominance of home care planning by either group. Considerable reasonableness was evidenced in patients', families', and professionals'
plans. Consequently, whose views of hypothetical home care needs
should be used to compare the costs of home and institutional care?

In the absence of strong evidence for or against control of home
care services by any of the three groups, and given the apparently
defensible positions of all, it may be possible to devise schemes
for home care planning to permit balanced influence by patients,
families, and various professionals. An appropriate balance would
be struck by granting precedence to group's views in ways which
draw on the strengths but circumscribe the weaknesses of each.

It is fortunate, for example, that professional agreement is clearly
worst in an area, household services, where patients and families
can be expected to have a good idea what they need. The latter
should therefore be permitted wide latitude in determining both
total hours of household help required, and how they should be
allocated among specific services and delivered by specific providers. Because of lingering suspicions of the inherent attractive-
ness of some household services to many persons, young and old,
public payers might demand that some sort of overall ceiling be
placed on spending. Professionals seem ill-equipped to perform this
task because of wide divergences in their views of needs for household services.

One step might be to set an absolute ceiling on the number of
hours of household help to be allowed all patients. Another would
be to validate need for household help in relation to objectively
measured functional ability and independence in instrumental activities of daily living. A considerable amount of research would
be required to learn the proper relationships: what constitutes too
much *or* too little overall help for different types of patients? Even
after such standards were in place, patients and their families might
be permitted to distribute the total among particular services. Thus,
a considerable measure of patient and family choice could be pre-
served even in the presence of valid and objective data.

A preferable way of validating household needs would consider
the impact on outcome, not only of services themselves, but the
process by which they were planned as well. Effects of professionally planned household services or of services allocated by
formula—in direct relation to objective patient characteristics—
might be compared with effects of services selected by patients

themselves—perhaps subject to the constraint that these cost no more than the first package. This procedure would measure the consequences for patient well-being of both the services and the planning process.

The desire to plan home care professionally or by formula (to plan *for* patients and families rather than *with* them) seems to stem from several motives: to be able to control, or at least predict, cost; to promote equity among patients; to allocate available resources in ways which do the most to enhance patient well-being; and, in some instances, to permit professionals to retain their present degree of influence over the home care planning process.

Fears of uncontrollable spending ensuing from patient or family influence over care planning find no support in the present study. Patients and families sought less paid help than professionals on average recommended. Patients, families, and professionals all seemed able to plan care equitably; professionals did a somewhat better job. About comparative effectiveness of the three sets of plans we know nothing.

In this context, experimentation with the process of care planning and the content of care plans, to learn what does the most for which patients, would be desirable. We need better knowledge of which method of care planning, involving more or less patient and family choice, best enhances outcomes for various patients. The same is required of the content of care itself. Better capacity to measure outcomes is a prerequisite for both.

The location of ultimate authority over the cost and content of home care must be fixed as part of any planning process. To satisfy legislators and administrators, authority will probably be granted to professionals operating within guidelines. The results of this study indicate, however, that allowing for patients or families a share of this authority would, on average, yield savings rather than cost increases. Therefore, in the absence of convincing evidence on the comparative effectiveness of plans prepared by the three groups and in the view of the possibility that consumer choice in long-term care enhances outcome, increased patient and family influence over planning for household and personal home care services should be permitted experimentally.

# PART III:
# SUPPORT FOR THE FAMILY

# Introduction to Part III

Part II of this collection assessed the demands that home care generates and the resources with which families try to cope with those demands. We saw that when the resources of families are not equal to the task, and when they do not receive help, the results can lead to inadequate care, or costly and unnecessary institutionalization, or deterioration and even breakdown in the family itself. We now approach these problems in social policy terms, shifting our perspective from the micro to the macro level and from the frustrations and rewards within families to the issues that confront society in caring for its dependent population.

Part III begins with a sweeping view of the changes that have taken place in American families and in the ways in which communities and society at large have responded to the needs of the physically dependent part of the population. From the viewpoint of an historian, Demos (below) reminds us that the meaning of dependency or vulnerability has changed as social and ecological conditions changed. For example, the elderly and the mildly retarded may not have been considered so dependent in earlier, simpler times when there were more opportunities for marginal work in an agricultural society. Beyond this, the values and attitudes in succeeding periods in our history have attached particular meanings to people who seemed alien, limited, "no longer fully human"—as has been the case with Indians, blacks, the physically deformed, and even children. Deep aversion has at times been the dominant feeling toward the vulnerable, whose "otherness" has evoked repugnance rather than empathy.

Another powerful influence that has shaped home care is the

American family itself, with all its variations over time and from one socioeconomic group to another. The composition and size of families, the sharpness of their boundaries, and the strength of affective ties have been much transformed from the early days of settlement in this country, through the Victorian period, and into this century.

One significant alteration, with direct impact on the care of dependent persons, has been the change in the functions performed by families. As an institution responsible for economic support, education, religious observance, and other tasks, the settlers' families were also responsible for care of the old, the sick, and the helpless. The community intervened only when these arrangements failed. The family of the 19th century, by contrast, was looked upon by many as an "island of peace," with many of its functions given over to specialized and professionalized institutions—among them the "asylums" where certain types of people could be both isolated from and cured of the effects of a disordered society.

Demos' tracing of change brings us to today's confusions about the role of families. Are they encounter-groups? Sources of acceptance, of excitement? If these define the family's role, Demos asks, what can be expected by way of sustained, committed responsibility to care for the dependent and disabled within the family?

One might anticipate that our laws—often the repository of the layers of changing attitudes and behavior which Demos describes—would define in clear terms the family's obligations to provide physical care and shelter to the disabled and the dependent. In fact, it is largely silent on these matters.* In law family responsibilities have for the most part been monetized or else defined in terms of avoidance of neglect. Nonetheless, as DeJong (below) and others have said, there is a general expectation that care will be given to a disabled and dependent person by relatives in the immediate family, with the State standing by to act when this expectation is not fulfilled. For the legal assumptions and precedents that bear on this inquiry, we must look to domestic relations law and legislation concerning support of relatives who are indigent and/or institutionalized.

The legal obligation of parents to provide care for their children

---

*The writer is indebted to Professor Mary Ann Glendon of the Boston College Law School and to Professor Saul Touster of Brandeis University for their assistance in exploring the legal aspects of this subject.

is the least uncertain of the lines of intra-familial responsibility. Here we find the concept of a minimum standard below which lies "neglect." Typically state statutes refer to "proper or necessary support," education, medical and other remedial care, or "other care as necessary" for the child's well-being (Krause, 1977, p. 236). Spouses, in the past often husbands but increasingly as a result of court decisions wives as well, are held liable for support in many states. The obligation that has been subject to the greatest erosion has been that of adult children toward their parents in financial need (Schorr, 1980; Lopes, 1975). It is reasonable to assume that the obligation to provide care to physically dependent relatives runs parallel to these definitions of relatives' responsibility for economic support.

A strong thrust toward relatives' responsibility in Anglo-Saxon law came in the 16th and 17th centuries and its motivation was fiscal and economic, the primary purpose being "to protect the public Purse" from the demands of an increasing body of poor people in England (Rosenbaum, 1967). The inclusion of the physically handicapped with the indigent is evident in this excerpt from the Poor Law of 1601:

> ". . . the father, grandfather, mother, grandmother, and children of every poor, old, blind, lame and impotent person or other person not able to work, being of sufficient ability shall at their own charges, relieve and maintain every such poor person according to the rate assessed by the justice of the peace." (Elizabeth 43)

The effort to save public funds by placing more of the financial burden on families has waxed and waned in the United States. Two examples illustrate a trend in recent decades to reverse the policy embodied in the English Poor Law. The 1965 amendments to the Social Security Act prohibited the imposition of family responsibility beyond spouse-for-spouse and parent-for-minor or disabled child (Acford, 1979). More recently when the Federal Government replaced the Old Age Assistance Program with the Supplemental Security Income program in 1974, the requirement of relative responsibility was eliminated from the statute.

These changes illustrate the general shift toward greater governmental responsibility, but the more recent surge of taxpayers' concern about the rising cost of social programs represents a coun-

tertrend that has the potentiality of tipping the seesaw back toward
the family as the primary locus of responsibility.

To summarize, the law clearly requires parents to provide minor
children with economic support, medical care, and other necessities
for their welfare, and much legislation and litigation in recent
years has reinforced these rights of children with regard to their
parents. It says little or nothing specifically about providing personal care to disabled, physically dependent relatives. Our laws
avoid directly compelling the rendering of personal services and
tend to formulate such obligations in terms of financial responsibility. The performance of services is not required, in part, because
this might damage relationships within the family.*

The silence of the law on this matter is not particularly significant since "Anglo-American family law is characteristically silent
on the details of on-going, functioning family life. Historically, it
comes into play only or mainly when family life is disrupted. The
silence of the law reflects the assumptions that . . . 'general care'
will be carried out voluntarily where possible, and that where it is
not being provided, there is little the law can or should do to
compel its provision *in kind*."** Social changes have been so continuous and so rapid in the past 100 years or even the last 50
years that the law has not been able to register a stable consensus
concerning the family's role in providing personal care.

Demos and Farber suggest that we are experiencing a rise in
individualism that emphasizes self-development and self-expression
and militates against the level of responsibility that physical care
of a disabled relative demands. But what appears as hedonism can
also be interpreted as the right to privacy and autonomy, well-
established in public policy especially since the 1930s in an elaborate structure of programs and services that relieve families of full
or even primary responsibility in many care-taking situations.

Glendon finds this de-emphasis on the family expressed in a
"gradual phasing out of the traditional unitary legal conception of
'the family.'"

> The convergence of the trends toward sex equality, free de-
> velopment of the individual personality, neutrality toward dif-
> ferent life-styles, and the blurring of distinctions between the

*Discussion with Prof. Touster
**Private communication from Prof. Glendon.

legitimate family and other types of families have had (so far as the law is concerned) the effect of concentrating on the individuals associated in families rather than on families as such. The nuclear family, so often said to be the "basic unit" of society, is now being broken down by the law and social programs into its component parts—the individual family members whom the law increasingly treats as separate and independent of each other. The individual as such is tending to be the unit of which the law takes account. (Glendon, 1981)

This is the same ideological shift to which Callahan refers when he writes of "individual entitlement" as a concept that "bestows certain rights on individuals independent of any responsibility on the part of family members." This was first expressed in social programs in this country in the initial provisions of the Social Security Act of the 1930s (Callahan et al., 1979, p. 1).

Clearly the locus of responsibility for caring for vulnerable people in American has shifted with time. For some years, this obligation seems to have been moving away from families, with the State conferring more benefits and entitlements on vulnerable and dependent individuals. But it is not clear from this formulation what is "cause" and what is "effect." Perhaps more important, our discussion has reached that junction between description and analysis on the one hand, and prescription and policy choice on the other hand. The question is not only where have we come from, but where do we want to go. Each direction that policy might take is closely related to an ideological position on the Welfare State. As Moroney poses the issues in his paper and in his more extensive writings on the subject, there are competing views (Moroney, 1976; Moroney, 1980):

(a) One can accept as desirable and/or inevitable the "fact" that families have progressively diminished the scope of their functions, including the caring role, and that it is appropriate for the State to expand its responsibilities accordingly to take up the slack left by the family's withdrawal.

(b) Our society rests on a strong family base and the tendency to reduce the responsibility of family members for each other should be resisted and reversed. Indeed, it is the very growth of the Welfare State and its proferring of assistance to its citizens that has encouraged families to withdraw from their legitimate duties toward their own members.

(c) The issue should not be dichotomized. The most socially sound approach is to assist families to maintain their efforts to provide home care for the dependent and this necessitates providing supportive services primarily through the resources of the State. The problem, according to this argument, is that services are so organized that they tend to substitute for the family and to supplant its efforts rather than supporting and assisting. This defeats a balanced approach that would simultaneously strengthen families, benefit dependent persons, and save billions of dollars.

Moroney argues the case for this last position. He looks upon family home care as a "vast social resource." He has found that families are in fact providing a "staggering amount" of care and that they want to provide that care. He concludes with this guide for policy:

> It would seem that in some situations families can provide better care and in others, the State would be the more appropriate caregiver. . . . The needs of families and individuals vary in time and over time and ideally the State would respond to these variations with policies that support families when they need support and substitute for families when they are incapable of meeting the needs of their members. Even this postulation is incomplete since it suggests a progression from no services to supportive services to substitute services, the last only when the family breaks down. In many cases a family may need some other social institution to temporarily assume the total caring function of a child or frail elderly parent but would reassume primary responsibility after the crisis has been dealt with. From this point of view, both functions (support and substitution) are necessary and neither can be offered as more important nor desirable than the other.

Have we, in actual practice, pursued such a policy? Most of the writing in this collection, especially the papers by Morell and Hart that follow, would suggest that we have not. Morell argues that with respect to mentally retarded children, the net effect of public decisions and actions has been to slow down the deinstitutionalization of these children and to deny their families the supportive help they require.

If policy in the field of mental retardation is judged by what is actually done, she argues, then a major obstacle to promoting family home care is the pattern of public expenditures. These have favored vocational training, employment opportunities and group homes for "retarded adults" at the expense of help to families with retarded children, for whom the existing services are inadequate to meet the real need. The second obstacle has been the overemphasis on the retarded person as the "client" rather than on "the provision of assistance to the family" who often needs relief from financial pressure, increased access to general social services, and additional options for short-term care.

Similar outcomes have occurred in home care of schizophrenics, Hart points out below. Here funding arrangements in both the public sector and in private insurance, as well as a lack of supportive services, have militated against care at home. The family, Hart observes, is victimized by contradictory policy impacts. "On the one hand, the financial support of the schizophrenic is supplemented during periods of hospitalization. On the other hand, prompt release and community care are encouraged but are not supported by the availability of appropriate facilities or by supplemental financial aid. One can deduce that while the patient is not hospitalized the family is left with the obligation of providing appropriate living arrangements as well as financial and social supports to the schizophrenic member." In addition, insurance benefits favor inpatient units of general hospitals over treatment in psychiatric hosptials and over partial hospitalization programs.

These two papers illustrate clearly the potential contribution that families can make to the care of the dependent and they expose the paucity of supports and services that are needed to sustain what Moroney has called "a vast social resource." Failing to receive such assistance, many families' resources are depleted, with serious consequences for all concerned. Indeed it is frequently the anticipation of either support or depletion that influences a family to undertake home care or shy away from it, as Segal (above) suggests. The availability of outside support and the terms on which it is offered are matters to which we now turn our attention.

Several lists have been compiled to indicate the kinds of services required to sustain family home care.* We have re-cast these into three categories in order to emphasize *the primary target* to whom they are addressed, as well as the *source* of the service: (1) services of a professional or technical nature given directly to the dependent person; (2) assistance that is given to the dependent person either by family members, unpaid friends and neighbors, or paid para-professionals; and (3) professional and paraprofessional services geared to the family to help its members discharge their care-taking roles. The list is intended to be suggestive of types of services, rather than exhaustive.

1. *Professional services for the dependent person*

>    Medical, dental, skilled nursing
>    Educational
>    Nutritional
>    Adult Day Care
>    Physical therapy
>    Speech therapy
>    Counseling
>    Orchestration of services
>    Advocacy
>    etc.

2. *Non-professional services for the dependent person*

>    Personal, bodily care
>    Psychological and social support
>    Companionship and/or "sitting"
>    Telephone reassurance
>    Recreation
>    Home-delivered meals
>    Transportation
>    Financial aid
>    etc.

3. *Supportive services for the family*

>    Home operation and maintenance (cooking, shopping, cleaning etc.)

---

*These include Callahan et al. 1978, p. 5; Gurland, 1978, p. 12; and Bruininks, 1979, pp. 4-7; HCFA, 1981, pp. 19-22. See Frankfather et al. 1981, pp. 34-35 for an analysis of services performed by families and the frequency of these activities.

Respite care
Social and psychological supports
Counseling and training
Financial assistance
etc.


Two cautions in using this list will be immediately apparent. First, some services can be placed in two or three categories. To illustrate, a physiotherapist may prescribe certain exercises but any responsible teenager or adult may be perfectly capable of helping the disabled person perform the exercises. In general, however, services can be identified as primarily in one classification or another. Secondly, it is not implied that all recipients of home care use or need all of these services and certainly not all of the time. The specifics in each case will vary with the physical condition, age, and other characteristics of the individual involved.

Overall, the literature reflects much less concern about the professional services used directly by the dependent person than it does about the other two categories. It is the partial or total lack of the simpler care-taking and family-maintaining assistance that is widely noted. Most of the writers in this collection repeatedly make the point that the inadequacy in these services is the main force that pushes families away from home care and toward the use of nursing homes, hospitals, and other institutions. A typical report is that given by Bruininks and his co-workers based on their study in six states:

> Parents, policy-makers and agency personnel indicated that family related services were both low in availability and quality. Nearly all the respondents indicated that incentives for care in the family home of a developmentally disabled person and respite care were not available or poor in quality. Furthermore, most of the respondents indicated a need for technical assistance in these areas. Interestingly, respondents to the survey felt that leisure, recreation, employment, and transportation services were particularly inadequate in availability and quality. (Bruininks, 1979, p. 4)

The reference above to respite care identifies one of the greatest gaps—the lack of a range of programs to take over the care takers' responsibilities for a limited amount of time.* For instance, to relieve a family from sleepless nights, a 24-hour, sleep-in aide would be helpful but is seldom available. Professor Moroney defined this as "short-term relief for the permanent care-taker." It may be carried out in or outside the home, for a few hours or for a one or two-week vacation period. He pointed out that in Britain 10 percent of nursing home placements are set aside for this purpose. Alternative arrangements include group care, such as a day care center for the frail elderly who would otherwise require nursing home placements. Western European countries in general have "much more extensive home help services than we do in the United States" (Kahn & Kamerman, 1975, Ch. 5).

Another instance of a mismatch between need and existing service is the agency requirement of a minimum number of hours of service. Generally homemakers and home health aides are provided by agencies for a minimum of four hours at a time. But it is often the case that a family needs someone to come in only to provide a meal or only to assist for an hour or two with personal care. The rigidity of the 4-hour rule results either in the denial of service because the family, in a sense, does not need enough help or in the provision of four hours of service when one or two are needed, with a consequent waste of resources and an indefensible cost that is borne either by the family or some public or private agency.

Another kind of rigidity in the present organization of services has to do with the sharp lines that are drawn to define "helping" roles. This was graphically illustrated by the account given by someone who had accompanied a social worker in London to see an old man who was physically handicapped and unable to get out of his apartment. The branches of a tree had been banging loudly against his window for weeks. The man wanted to have someone cut off the annoying branches. The social worker said this was not an appropriate request for him to handle, since it did not involve a professional service.

This incident prompted the question why there cannot be a simple system to provide people like the man in the London flat with a specific amount of money, perhaps on a formula basis. The individual would determine how to use the funds. The man in London could have spent it in a way that was quite unique to him,

---

*The observations in the next few pages are from the discussions among consumers, providers, and academics at the conference which is identified in the Acknowledgments.

to meet a need that no one else could have anticipated. He would have been able to hire someone to do what was necessary with the tree that was banging on his window incessantly.

In this country much of the outside assistance comes from three types of workers. *Home health aides* are usually employed by an agency such as a Visiting Nurse Association and are assigned in accordance with a doctor's treatment plan. The aide takes care of bathing, dressing, grooming, toliet care, and the like. Under certain conditions, Medicare and Medicaid will pay for a home health aide. *Homemakers,* usually in the employ of a home care, family, or proprietary agency, and *chore workers,* who are usually hired by the dependent person, do light housekeeping but not much personal care. Homemakers and chore workers can be paid for under Title XX of the Social Security Act. There has been some experimentation with attendant care workers (or Personal Care Attendants) also employed directly by the client, who perform both personal care tasks and light housekeeping; Medicaid and Title XX can support attendant care.

There are important strictures in these programs which discourage home care (HCFA, 1981, p. 19; U.S. DHEW, 1978). Medicare's "skilled care" requirement precludes persons who need only "less skilled" supportive care and its "homebound" requirement may discourage a patient from returning home from an institution. Moreover, there is no provision in Medicare for supportive services "related to the needs of daily living, such as homemaker or nutrition services, which are often necessary to prevent institutionalization."

Medicaid spends less than three percent of its long-term care funds on home health care, primarily because of its spend-down provision which means that many persons become eligible only after incurring large medical expenses, "almost always as a result of some form of institutional care." Ironically, the costs of in-home services under most circumstances would not be great enough to establish eligibility for Medicaid. The HEW report further criticizes Medicare and Medicaid regulations for making it unattractive for service providers to participate, thus restricting supply. As for Title XX, the quality of care is said to be often inadequate, with anecdotal evidence of "appalling instances of low quality care."

When a paraprofessional does come into a home, what can be done is often as circumscribed as we found it to be in the incident in London. If one's function, for example, is defined narrowly as physical care, to the exclusion of developing a friendly relationship, the assistance is only partial. On the other hand, as Professor Moroney pointed out in the conference, homemakers who are encouraged not just "to do the dirty work and then leave," quickly come to value "talking" more than giving physical care, a situation that has arisen in England. This calls for more careful training and supervision. But this in turn, Professor Morris noted, is one of the reasons that 50-75 percent of the cost of homemaker and home health services goes for administration rather than direct service.

Another problematic area concerns the skills of the family and the vulnerable person. If they could be better trained in caretaking techniques, both would be better able to cope. But such training, which can contribute to greater independence on the part of the disabled person, is often lacking.

Finding and retaining paid personnel presents its own problems. Pay scales are usually too low to attract people to this kind of employment. Suggestions were made about employing young people, especially from the large pool of unemployed young men. Two difficulties were noted: attitudes concerning personal care of women by men and the suitability of young people as aides to the aged. Both positive and negative experiences were reported.

Ineligibility for existing benefits because a family exceeds the permissible income level is a major barrier to home care. Those who are eligible for Medicaid or Medicare benefits get some help, however inadequate it may be. But the market fails those families who are just above the income limits and who are hard-pressed to pay the full cost of services. Families farther up in the middle class apparently have evolved an "entrepreneurial" model of help-seeking, in which they avoid public agencies and locate their own sources of assistance. In this context it was also reported that some families of developmentally disabled persons have almost totally rejected professional help and have opted instead for a system of self-help. One of the reasons for this may be that these families show little tendency to proceed in terms of a medical model, that is, they do not operate on the assumption that there is a "cure" for their dependent family member.

There is another way in which families turn out to be ineligible for financial assistance with home care—they are defined out by insurance plans, as Hart (below) explains. Current practices offer financial assistance to a schizophrenic while he or she is hospitalized, but withhold aid when the patient is at home. Hart also shows that the way in which schizophrenia is defined (i.e., as a medical problem or an "interactional disturbance") determines the sources of help, the kind of help, and often the amount.

This brief review of home care services has indicated where the critical issues lie, issues which left unresolved can jeopardize a large, informal system of family-based service. These include a stark lack of certain services such as respite care; the provision of some services that are judged to be poor in quality; rigidities in the delivery system that make assistance to families more remote; and income restrictions that exclude families who are above the officially designated low income line but who still face onerous financial and non-material costs. The existing public regulations, furthermore, appear to discourage providers from offering services. Operating singly or in combination these factors have the effect of tilting families away from home care and toward institutional care.

These, moreover, are some of the practical issues that bedevil the difficult policy choices, considered in Part IV, that must be made in coping, socially and politically, with the needs of dependent persons and their families.

# Family Home Care:
# Historical Notes and Reflections

## John Demos

Our subject is a large one and its historical context is much
larger still. The chronological limits of this presentation will be
nothing less than the full range of American history. The viewpoint from which I will survey this range will be that of the
family. I will attempt, in short, to relate questions of care for
vulnerable persons to "family history." Along the way I will propose a little scheme for periodizing the field—a model of family
history, if you will.

## I.

Before getting to the substance of all this, I want to propose
something else, which emerges very quickly from any historical
review of the topic before us. It is necessary, I think, to recognize
as clearly as possible a variety of relevant factors—"dimensions"
might be a better word—in which change through history is possible, or likely, or even (in some cases) inevitable. Let me offer a
short list of the ones which strike me as being especially important.

There is, first, the matter of *cultural context,* insofar as it bears
directly on the status of the vulnerable person—and indeed on the
idea of vulnerability itself. In part, this involves implicit or explicit definitions current within a given historical population: what
circumstances, and what individuals, are most readily associated
with vulnerability? In part, too, it reflects social and ecological
realities. Perhaps, for example, in pre-modern times the elderly
and the mildly retarded were more favorably positioned than is
the case nowadays. On the one hand, the round of their daily
experience was simpler and more manageable; on the other, the
local economy offered opportunities for marginal work (e.g., some
aspects of horticulture; handicrafts; child care) which lay within
their limited capacities. To that extent at least some of them may

have felt—and may actually have been—less vulnerable than their counterparts of our own day.

A second set of considerations, no less important, has a *demographic and biomedical foundation*. The absolute numbers of the vulnerable, and their proportion within the larger population to which they belong: these things, too, are very much subject to change. All pre-modern communities experienced high levels of mortality and morbidity—high, that is, by our own standards. And these, in turn, particularly affected persons who were born with incapacities or had acquired them through subsequent experience. The numerical ratios as between different categories of vulnerability have also varied over time. Nowadays, for example, the elderly comprise a substantial part of the entire "vulnerable" population—whereas two or three centuries ago they were comparatively few (and quite possibly were healthier, on average, than their modern counterparts). By the same token, young children were severely at risk in an earlier time; while now their vulnerability, at least in a biological sense, is less than that of most older age-groups. Finally, we must reckon with the numbers and status of the potential caretakers—those best situated to look after their vulnerable culture-mates. It is a commonplace of discussion on this topic that the caretaker pool is just now undergoing a drastic reduction—given the massive movement of adult women into the labor force.

The third entry on my list of historically variable "dimensions" is more subtle—and far more difficult to specify. But, simply stated, the fate of the vulnerable is influenced by "soft" undercurrents of normative structure and psychological disposition, no less than by the "hard facts" of social or demographic process. Some of this is open and visible: vulnerability itself may be scorned, or tolerated, or even (in some circumstances) glorified. One thinks in this connection of certain characteristic values of "Victorian" America—a whole ethos of sympathy and tenderness that flowered in the middle of the last century. (I must add, parenthetically, that this was a very two-sided situation; for along with the tenderness went a new cult of toughness, a quest for *in*vulnerability.) Other elements are hidden from view; they reach indeed into depth psychology. The capacity to respond empathically to conditions of need is unevenly distributed among individuals—likewise among whole generations or cultures. This variance depends, in turn, on the scope and shape of self/other distinctions. I have argued elsewhere that old people in early America suffered from deeply aversive attitudes in the not-old. To be elderly was to be alien, strange, no longer fully human. "Otherness," in general, was poorly comprehended and little appreciated—witness the prevalent ideas among the "settlement" generations about Indians, blacks, and even their own children. Some of this pattern has survived to the present day, in at least attenuated forms. I am struck, for example, at the discomfort—even repugnance—experienced by many "normal" persons nowadays in the presence of others with overt physical handicaps. And I would speculate that this reaction was less common and less powerful among pre-modern peoples. Firm evidence on such points is lacking, but we should assume no unilinear trends or tendencies.

A fourth important "dimension" includes the many forms of organized social response: public and private, large and small, voluntary and coercive, institutional and/or supportive (e.g., "outdoor relief"). It is widely supposed that "government"—in one form or another—has taken an increasingly large share of the responsibility for vulnerable persons—with a corresponding diminution in the role of families. This will need substantive consideration—both in the present paper, and also, I suspect, in those that follow.

Fifth—and finally—there is the dimension of *family* itself. The composition of families, the sharpness and strength of their boundaries, the nature of their internal structures, their affective arrangements, the image and expectations which define them for their constituent members: here is still another large territory of potential change. Indeed, as I've already announced, it is from within this territory that I plan to launch the historical forays which will comprise the rest of this paper.

## *II.*

My rendition of American family history divides, like Caesar's Gaul, into three parts. Part One begins with the beginning—that is, with the various European settlements made on our shores early in the seventeenth century—and continues for nearly 200 years. Part Two runs from the opening decades of the nineteenth century until the middle of the twentieth. And Part Three is us, or at least some of us: where we are, and where we seem likely to be going. I trust you will excuse the looseness of this periodization;

obviously investigations of this sort cannot be made to yield precise chronological markings. Each stage overlaps the others, and the entire process is cumulative. Moreover, exceptions could readily be found for every part of the model; we are dealing at best with overall *tendencies*.

The first stage comprises patterns of family life to which some historians apply the general term "pre-modern." A central feature was the evident permeability—one might also say the complementarity—of the individual family vis-à-vis the community at large. Families were seen as the building blocks from which all larger units of social organization could be fashioned. A family was itself a little society, exemplifying the same principles that prevailed in villages, colonies, nations, and empires. Experience within and without would, under normal circumstances, be continuous. The family performed a multitude of functions, both for its individual members and for the aggregate to which it belonged. Thus most of what children received by way of formal education was centered around the home hearth; likewise their training in particular vocations, in religious worship, and in what we would call "good citizenship." Illness was also a matter of home care: I don't need to tell you that there was no hospital system in early America. Society at large—represented by duly constituted civil authorities—maintained a position of oversight on the welfare of families. And when there was malfunction of one sort or another, the authorities did not hesitate to intervene. Thus the courts might order a married couple to "live more peaceably together" or to upgrade the "governance" of their children. Failure to respond to such orders could result in more forcible intervention, and even in punishment such as fines or whippings.

And how, specifically, were vulnerable persons affected by all this? I have already alluded to children and their biological vulnerability (especially during their first years); here, for certain, was a major area of family responsibility. Young children were cared for by their own parents (or step-parents), sometimes with the important but temporary assistance of a wet nurse. Only occasionally was this care deemed insufficient by the standards of the time; but the exceptions are worth at least passing notice. When a particular child seemed not to be receiving adequate care, local authorities would act—usually to remove him (or her) from the family of origin and place him in another family. Most such cases involved children judged to be living "in idleness," or without appropriate discipline; in a sense, therefore, their vulnerability was moral. A few older children, already bound out as servants or apprentices, were found to have suffered physical abuse (another form of vulnerability); they, too, would be sent by official order from one household to another. There is little direct evidence of children suffering from physical, mental, or emotional handicap, but this is because they remained with their own families, entering no wider orbit of concern. Occasionally one does find a will or a deed of gift, which makes special reference to a son or daughter "disenabled" (in one case) by "the lameness of his hand" or (in another) by "the weakness of her reason and understanding." Such persons might receive extra bequests of property—and, when they proved completely "uncapable," the responsibility for them would be transferred to siblings or other relatives.

The mention of other relatives calls to mind a hoary shibboleth of historical sociology: the so-called "extended family" once thought to have been an integral part of pre-modern society. This notion has been largely discredited by much recent research, but it may need a little further discrediting—specifically in the present context. We must not imagine that the care of vulnerable persons was, in bygone days, managed through an extended-family system. For there was no extended-family system at any point in Western history (or at least for as far back as the evidence allows us to see). Instead, nuclear families seem always to have been the norm. More remotely related kin were drawn into the care of the vulnerable only when the members of the immediate family had died or disappeared. Indeed we can draw up a rank order of responsibility on exactly this point. Parents were the primary caretakers, so long as they were able; then siblings; then grandparents; then aunts, uncles, cousins. Lacking any relatives in all these categories (and occasionally even when some *were* available), the vulnerable person became the charge of civil authorities. The usual result in such cases was his assignment to some other family in the community.

Similar principles applied in the care of the elderly. Most elderly persons preferred to look after themselves for as long as they could, and many succeeded in doing so to an advanced age. Of course, an individual—or a couple—rendered aged *and* infirm needed special help. Sometimes there was a formal transaction involving the exchange of property (from the old folks) for regular care (by the young folks); usually this meant some sort of joint living arrangement. Often such arrangements were managed *in-formally*. But the key point is that most of them followed blood lines: typically the aged-infirm wound up in the household of someone among their grown children. The pattern is most vividly represented for us by probate documents. Countless wills and estate settlements record elaborate provision for the care of the testator's *widow*. For widows, it seems, were inherently more vulnerable than their male counterparts. Most vulnerable of all, however, were those among the aged who lacked health, material resources, *and* children (or other family) living nearby. With them, once again, the civil center of the community served as the last line of protection. Local records throughout the colonies display a variety of substantive ways and means for dealing with such cases. In effect, they add up to "outdoor relief": provisions and services delivered piecemeal, more or less as need warranted.

We must notice one final point about the early American pattern. There was, by our lights at least, a certain lack of discrimination among the various kinds of vulnerability. The term "poor" served to cover a broad range of conditions—poverty, to be sure, but also infirmity, old age, specific types of handicap, and even an absence of kin. To be "poor" meant simply to stand in need. This usage mattered little so long as most vulnerable persons remained in domestic settings—cared for by those who knew their particular wants and problems from long personal experience. It was of greater consequence, however, when a new, "institutional" mode of response began to emerge. The first colonial "almshouses" and "workhouses" were established during the middle of the eighteenth century in a few urban centers like Boston, New York, and Philadelphia. The inmate population was a mixed bag of indigence, infirmity, insanity, orphanage, and old age—in varying amounts and combinations. To this group were sometimes added derelicts, habitual drunkards, and outright criminals. The numbers involved were at first very small; the vast majority of vulnerable persons continued to be found in household settings. But this served, all the same, as the harbinger of a new—and considerably different—future.

We must now take a great leap forward, right out of the colonial period and into the brave new world of the nineteenth century. For here beginneth the second part of American family history.

Briefly, a few essential stage-props: The country has launched itself on a career of "independence," and the people embrace new goals, new precepts, a new cultural identity. According to a loudly voiced consensus, America has thrown off the shackles of traditional society; the barriers of rank and privilege are down; life is a race, open to talent, with "success" as the ultimate prize. Growth and newness pervade the land; "improvement" is Everyman's watchword, and "the go-ahead spirit" keeps him moving relentlessly forward. Commerce expands enormously; industry makes a strong beginning. At the center of all this are the cities— the older ones of the seaboard, and then, increasingly, the new ones of the midwest. There, in the urban melting pot, the swift currents of change converge in a roil of creative ferment.

To the people directly involved this process seems alluring, exciting, liberating, in some respects—but deeply frightening, in others. Some of the currents are dark and dangerous. Cherished ways are going under, to be replaced by—what? By greed, by deceit, by ruthless competitive striving. There is a growing sense of bearings lost and values betrayed.

Against this cultural backdrop domestic life is redefined. Household composition does not much change (husband, wife, children, plus an occasional servant or lodger), but the family itself acquires new meaning. Within the gathering maelstrom "Home" holds firm—or so it is hoped—an island of peace, a little citadel where the old virtues still have their due. The boundaries are clearly drawn, the portals carefully guarded. Home is no longer one community among many; its morale, its purposes, and its social importance are special. Home and "the world"—Home *versus* "the world"—these are now separate "spheres," with opposite styles and values. The predominant theme of home life becomes protection. Here, in particular, the wife/mother and her children are shielded from the grinding pressures and dark temptations of society at large. Here, too, the husband/father periodically takes cover from the bitter struggles of the workplace, the marketplace, and the political arena.

In a sense everyone is vulnerable now. And the giving and receiving of *care* is virtually synonymous with domestic experience. Of course, home has always been a caring place; but in nineteenth-century America this equation is intensified and made explicit as never before. And what is its bearing on the situation of vulnerable persons—not simply the morally imperiled, but those who cannot fully look after themselves from day to day?

The enormous growth of institutional settings throughout the first half of the nineteenth century is a sign of new forces at work. Mental hospitals, almshouses, orphanages, old age homes—along with penitentiaries and reformatories: such places sprout by the dozens across the land. These "asylums"—as they are collectively termed—express a new set of social attitudes. Insanity—for one example—and poverty—for another—are now related to social causes. In the colonial period each of these conditions was incorporated into a "providential" world-view; each was seen as belonging to God's plan and will. In the nineteenth century, by contrast, insane persons are treated as casualties of excessive stress and excitement in the environment. Poor folk, meanwhile, are thought to have suffered for their own moral failings—here is our ancient tradition of "blaming the victim"—yet "worldly temptation" is usually cited as a proximate cause. Considered overall, dependency is both a symptom and an effect of social disorder—and it threatens to become a cause of further disorder. The appropriate response is, therefore, to isolate the individuals involved. Only thus can they be "reformed"; and only thus can a truly massive contamination be averted.

The place of the family, within this framework of understandings, is quite critical. Simply stated: dependency frequently implies *domestic* no less than social disorder—the family has failed in its nurturing and protective functions. Hence "outdoor relief" can serve only to perpetuate the problem; hence, again, the "asylum." In specific cases the family becomes the enemy of the asylum—and of the reform which the asylum promises. Here is an actual expression of this viewpoint taken from the records of the Baltimore House of Refuge. The date is 1857; the words are those of the House superintendent:

> Only two weeks ago there were three applications for the discharge of children. We refused upon this ground: we did not think it proper, under the charter, that the parents should obtain the committal of their children, and after two or three months, upon the application of the same individual who made the commitment, the child should be given up. . . . You cannot expect reform in under two years. The managers must have complete power over the child until he has attained the age of twenty-one. He finds that there is no hope of speedy discharge, submits to the discipline, and improves. . . . (Another) case recently occurred which may serve to illustrate

the advantage of guardianship till majority. Two very interesting children, a girl and a boy, were sent to us last winter.
Being extremely destitute, they were committed as vagrants,
and we took charge of them. After we had found a home for
the little girl, the mother made an application for her, which
we refused. . . . She threatened legal proceedings, but our
power over the child was superior to hers, and thus the
injudicious interference of the parents was prevented . . .

"The injudicious interference of parents was prevented"—let that
phrase sink in. In fact, the operating procedure of insane asylums
usually follows a similar premise. Thus a Pennsylvania asylum ad-
vises would-be visitors that "the visits of strangers among the
patients are often much less objectionable than those of friends
or relatives"; as for the immediate family, "the welfare of the
patient often demands that they should be completely interdicted."

These materials suggest a clear clash of interest and purpose,
as between the institution, on the one hand, and the inmate's
family, on the other. Yet are there no instances where the two
sides may cooperate? At least occasionally, perhaps, the family
is more than willing to accept the institutionalization of one of
its members. Perhaps the financial costs of caring for an elderly
grandmother are too great. (The family has its own prospects to
consider—and there is a church-sponsored "home for the aged"
just over town.) Perhaps the emotional costs of looking after a
disturbed child become unbearable. (Home, after all, must be kept
as a place of good order—and the youngster's antics are most
unsettling. Placement in the local House of Refuge will be a
benefit to all concerned.)

However, we must not imagine that huge numbers of vulnerable
persons are now being hurried into institutions by their families
and kept there by overzealous superintendents. Surely the great
majority of them remain in the care of relatives. In practice, most
inmates of nineteenth-century asylums either (1) have no family
available to them, or (2) come from "the dregs of society" (a
favorite period phrase) where family life carries a presumption of
failure. It is no coincidence, for example, that immigrants and
unskilled laborers (and their children) are disproportionately represented in these places. Families above the lowest class, and WASP
families generally, still manage—by and large—to look after their
own.

What seems most novel, and potentially significant, about these nineteenth-century developments is a new balance of interests around the vulnerable person. In some respects his own interest appears to clash with that of his family. In others the clash is between his family and the asylum. It is no longer clear that a familial setting is best for all parties, and that extrafamilial involvement should (with infrequent exceptions) be limited to piecemeal support.

The family as community, the family as refuge: these notions are part of our legacy from the past, and they retain considerable vitality today. And yet our sense of family is changing once again—in ways that reverberate to many corners of our experience. As a caption for the new mode I submit: "the family as encounter group." For the central values attaching to domestic experience nowadays, at least as I read them, are indeed those which underscore significant personal encounters.

The context of this change is a lessening of the sense of social threat—which was so fundamental to the nineteenth-century image—and the growth of a new complaint. Life in the world outside Home now seems merely monotonous, as, increasingly, experience comes to us in standardized chunks. There is a grayness, a flatness, a sameness about the "mass society" in which we are all caught up. I am running through some buzz-words here so that it won't be necessary to ring all the changes on what is certainly a familiar theme.

The implication specifically for family life seems to be this: Since our individuality counts for so little in work and in civic life generally, we bring to personal relationships a special set of compensatory needs. We look to our spouses, our lovers, even our children, to make us feel alive and affirmed. A good relationship, we say, is one in which both parties "grow"—whatever their age and status. This modish invocation of personal "growth" reflects very sharply our altered expectations of family. For "growth" would be unlikely where Home served primarily as a refuge. The contrast between the nineteenth- and the twentieth-century images is most instructive. *Then* Home was to be a place of peace and repose; *now* it must generate some excitement. *Then* roles, rights, and responsibilities within Home were shaped to an overall model of harmony; now they are measured in terms of personal enhancement. I am deliberately overstating my argument here. A good deal of the old way survives, yoked uncomfortably to the new one; but the difference overall seems unmistakable.

And now, one more time, the matter of vulnerable family members. Demographic change and structural change have created some new—or at least altered—equations. The elderly, for example, are an increasingly sizable group in relation to the population at large; and long life-expectation (on average), together with lowered birth rates, argue against any reversal of this trend in the foreseeable future. Moreover, the heroic procedures of modern medicine preserve many lives despite severe injury and incapacity—lives which, in an earlier time, would have been greatly foreshortened. To this extent the pool of vulnerable persons seems enlarged.

At the opposite end of the life cycle, the picture looks quite different. We have fewer and fewer children to look after, and the ones we do have are literally immune to the ancient scourges of epidemic disease. However, handicap of one sort or another—now largely derived "from birth"—is a considerable presence among our young; and, again, the effect of medical science is to increase the size of this most affectingly vulnerable subgroup. There is also a sense, I think, in which all children are more vulnerable now than their counterparts in generations gone by. On the one hand, they can no longer serve any productive function; on the other, their education—and their "rearing" in general—is a long, complex, and expensive process. In our cost-conscious society the price tag on child-rearing has become a lively subject of interest; some estimates go as high as $100,000 per kid. When parents are unable or unwilling to pay this price, the children involved are very much at risk.

There is one specific token of the increased vulnerability of the young: the much-lamented but clearly widespread problem of child abuse. I want to record here my own impression that child abuse—understood to mean injurious physical assault by adults on their own offspring—is a relatively modern phenomenon. I know that some opinion runs the other way. It seems easier to believe that children of the past were as much (or more) subject to abuse—and that societies of the past didn't even care. Easier to believe, but I think wrong. The pressures that lead to abuse seem stronger now, and the constraints are generally weaker; and the results offer a keen reproach to our own social system.

To be sure, most present-day parents do not abuse their children; but there are additional grounds for concern that may have a much wider application. There is child neglect: physical neglect, emotional neglect, or some combination of the two. More significant still is a growing vein of skepticism about the very idea of parenthood. Roughly two centuries ago American parents began trying for the first time to limit the numbers of their offspring; and roughly two generations ago they gained the means to effect such limitation about as they wished. And now we have another historic first: a decision by some portion of adults not to rear children at all. (I am reminded of an article in the *New York Times Magazine* a few years ago. The authors, a married couple, had recently produced a child. Virtually none of their friends and acquaintances had thought to take this novel step; hence their own experience seemed both newsworthy and in need of lengthy justification!)

The reasons for rejecting parenthood are no doubt quite various; but there is, all the same, an underlying melody. Children—it is said—are so needy, so vulnerable in the sense of requiring care and guidance and protection, that their parents have little opportunity to "grow." The values of self-enhancement simply conflict—and finally take precedence. Of course, it can be argued that parenting is itself a "growth experience"; but much depends on the circumstances. Perhaps we should take a positive view of all this: presumably, it is good that people who do not want children should not have them in the first place. And yet there is another view, at least as plausible and considerably more ominous. For every adult who decides against parenthood, there may be a dozen more who undertake it ambivalently—or, at some level, unwillingly. The aforementioned value conflicts can hardly be confined to the childless. Indeed the decision (by some) not to parent may well signify a sea-change in social attitudes—a new indifference, if not an outright aversion, toward vulnerability in all its shapes and guises.

Lest the drift of this presentation become overly bleak, I must mention also some countertendencies. Consider, for example, the whole idea of social insurance, and its various forms of programmatic expression. Pension plans, the social security system, workmen's compensation, even programs like the oft-maligned AFDC: these relatively recent developments weigh strongly on the side of ameliorative response to vulnerability. More than that, they have positive implications for family care of vulnerable persons. (Professor Moroney has carefully explored these implications in his very useful book *The Family and the State*.) The current situation of the aged is instructive. The fact that elderly people have financial support from extra-familial sources—social security, retirement income, or whatever—may actually enhance their prospects of receiving intra-family care. Something of the same effect can be expected from a program of national health insurance in the (hopefully) near future. I should also like to notice, in this connection, a proposal for "Childhood Disability Insurance" advanced in the recent report of the Carnegie Council on Children. The purpose of such a scheme would be to insure parents against the disproportionate costs of rearing a handicapped child. Its effect— and part also of its purpose—would be to alter the balance of choice as between family care and long-term institutionalization.

The point of all such schemes, of course, is to limit the financial burdens imposed on families by the care of vulnerable persons. Yet the burdens are never exclusively financial ones. Right here I wish to return to the matter of the expectations which we characteristically bring to family life. When these expectations run so strongly to "growth," to personal fulfillment, even to "liberation," the responsibility for day-by-day care of others may become a source of intolerable frustration. The goals of inward self and the realities of interpersonal obligation are set on a collision course from which there can be no easy escape. I do not mean to suggest that any part of this situation is easy—or contrived—or false; nor do I wish to render moral judgment on those involved. We are all children of our time and culture, and we certainly cannot move ourselves into new attitudes by simple efforts of exhortation. Here I find myself in substantial agreement with a recent statement by Professor Bernard Farber.

May I quote:

> The current world-view with which we operate informs us that increasingly technology and modernization of culture have brought a large measure of control over our environment. For a measure of social progress we look to history, and history does reveal many effects of modernization—such as increase in length of life, heightening of quality of life, and greater realization of human potentiality. The decline in infant mortality, the virtual elimination of epidemics, and the decreases in widespread famine—all of these lend support to the perspective that we are progressively gaining control over those elements which are destructive to human life and society. . . . The media of mass communication and mass entertainment promise immediate, no-cost gratification, civil rights for all, instant success, a cure for every illness and

an illness for every cure. The notion that all deficiencies can somehow be remedied implies that someone—usually a professional specialist—is available to remove whatever impedes the American dream.

Professor Farber calls attention to the central values of our cultural macrocosm. I would like to emphasize—actually, to *re*-emphasize—the presence of such values in the domestic *micro*cosm. The family as encounter group: how can the vulnerable person be fitted *there*?

## *III.*

I have taken you on a long—and, I fear, rather arduous—historical journey. Perhaps, in conclusion, it would be helpful to recall just where we have been.

We began by visiting the first two centuries of American history. There we discovered vulnerable people mostly in the care of their own families. When that arrangement didn't serve, they were moved to other families—usually on the orders of civil authority. The role of authority was generally supportive, and at least occasionally support took the form of "outdoor relief." The entire pattern seemed, at least from this distance, relatively smooth and conflict-free.

Next, we toured the nineteenth century, viewing the deep causes and vast effects of "modernization." We noticed, in particular, a new development directly affecting the fate of the vulnerable—the growth of a panoply of "asylums." Still, the family remained by all odds the principal source of care. Seen whole, the situation displayed a new complexity: the interests of the family, of the asylum, and of the vulnerable person were sometimes in conflict.

Finally, we looked at where we are now. Families continue, in the great majority of cases, to provide for their own—with institutions as the obvious alternative. But the size and shape of the vulnerable population is significantly altered. Social insurance has helped to reduce the costs of care—and may actually sustain intra-family arrangements. But there are additional costs and burdens which are not so easily confronted. In particular, there is confusion and conflict deriving from our current value system. The wish to help is far from disappearing; but it clashes, in practice, with other wishes, other aspirations. There is little reason to think that the clash will soften in the future; indeed some signs point the other way.

But I will not try to follow these signs. Like most historians' time machines, mine has no forward gear . . .

# A Legal Perspective on Disability, Home Care, and Relative Responsibility

## Gerben DeJong

Public policy has been most ambiguous toward the role of relatives in providing in-home assistance to a disabled person. One branch of thinking asserts that caring for a disabled person is the natural responsibility of relatives who should perform the caring function without compensation. Another branch of thinking argues that family care is a precarious but needed source of care and should be compensated, in part, to reduce the reliance on more expensive forms of institutional care. Public ambiguity on this subject stems from a long-standing moral and legal tradition regarding the role of relatives in the care and maintenance of their disabled and elderly kin.

The matter of relative responsibility has been left almost entirely to the states.[1] However, state laws have been largely silent on the specific issue of relative responsibility for home health and personal care. Therefore, it is necessary to go outside the area of home care policy to consider how state statutes and the courts have defined relative responsibility in other areas of social policy. While state laws have not been explicit about relative responsibility in home care, state agency policies governing home care programs are guided by the assumptions and requirements of relative responsibility statutes that apply to three areas: domestic relations, income maintenance, and institutional care. These legal assumptions and requirements often go unchallenged when incorporated into a state's home care policies. This paper seeks to identify these assumptions and requirements and to determine the extent to which they are or should remain normative in state home care policy for disabled persons.

This paper was supported in part by grant #G008200039 from the National Institute of Handicapped Research, Department of Education, Washington, D.C. 20202.

While focusing on the assumptions and requirements of relative responsibility statutes, we also want to determine:

—Whether relatives are, in fact, legally liable to provide or pay for the care of disabled persons in their own homes: and,
—Whether relatives can be compensated from public sources for the care they provide a disabled family member.

No litigation appears to have reached the appellate level challenging federal and state policies with respect to the role of relatives in providing home care for a disabled person. The absence of litigation belies the amount of discontent among home care consumers. For example, severely physically disabled persons often remain unmarried in order to retain their eligibility for income maintenance and medical assistance benefits, or in order to allow their mates to be compensated for the attendant care he or she provides. Some consumers consider it a serious injustice when a nonrelative can be paid for the very same care that a spouse can provide but cannot be compensated.

In the absence of specific litigation on the issue of relative responsibility and home care, what then are the legal assumptions and requirements that have informed the formation of policy in this area? Is there any way to predict how the courts are likely to rule if such an issue did arise? Has there been litigation in related areas that might serve as a guide as to how the relative responsibility issue would be resolved in the home care area? Can some evolution in thinking on the relative responsibility issue be discerned?

The legal assumptions and requirements that inform this area of public policy arise out of two legal traditions: (1) family law, and (2) poor law. Within the poor law tradition, the issue of relative responsibility has arisen in two subareas: (a) income maintenance, particularly in the care of aged parents, and (b) institutional care, particularly in the care of mentally disabled persons.

## *FAMILY LAW*

Family law prescribes the responsibilities between members of the nuclear family—between husband and wife and between parents and children. The rules that comprise family law are backed by a long tradition of religious teachings and moral precepts. In the English legal tradition the duties between husband and wife were considered reciprocal: the husband was to provide the family with food, clothing, shelter, and other amenities while the wife was to maintain the home and care for the children.[2] Failure to live up to their responsibilities brought the intervention of either the civil or ecclesiastical courts.

The English model was adopted almost in its entirety in colonial America. The principle of husband support is largely a matter of common law,[3] although states have statutes requiring a husband to support his wife.[4] A good number of states have Family Expense Acts which require both parties to support the family. The wording of these statutes varies widely but their thrust is that expenses of the family are chargeable against the property of both husband and wife.[5] Some states impose no personal liability on the wife but merely impose a liability against property owned while married.[6]

At common law there appears to have been no legal obligation on the father's part to support his children.[7] However, statutes relating to the maintenance of poor persons did impose such an obligation, as we shall see in our discussion on the poor laws.[8] Today, the father is primarily liable for the support of his children,[9] with the mother liable if he fails or refuses to provide support.[10]

One method of enforcing child support is to allow a mother or child to purchase "necessaries" and charge them to the father. Another method is to have the child bring civil suit against the father in order to acquire periodic support payments. The "doctrine of necessaries" is not limited to the purchase of basic necessities as the term suggests. Necessaries are defined to be those goods and services that take into account individual needs, the father's income, and the family's socioeconomic status. Thus, the father can be made liable for medical and dental expenses as well as food, clothing, and shelter.[11]

All states make nonsupport of children a criminal offense, and nearly all states also make nonsupport of wives a criminal offense.[12] Most states treat the offense as a misdemeanor and sometimes as a felony with a maximum sentence of three years.[13] A few states also provide criminal penalties for parents who fail to support an incapacitated adult child[14] or for wives who fail to support an incapacitated husband.[15]

To summarize, family law governs the behavior of members within the nuclear family. It reinforces the moral obligation of spouses to support one another and of parents to support children. The law is less clear as to what exactly constitutes support beyond ordinary food, clothing, and shelter. The doctrine of necessaries strongly suggests that personal care and basic household maintenance are activities that come within the meaning of family support. These obligations are backed by legal sanctions in the form of criminal penalties. Thus, it would appear that spouses, especially husbands, are legally liable to provide or arrange the home care services they or their children may need.

The legal liability of spouses or parents to provide basic in-home care does not prevent the state or any of its agencies from providing or supplementing the care a spouse or parent may furnish. It does, however, give state agencies the right to exclude potential recipients of home care services unless other statutes specifically prohibit such an exclusion.

## *POOR LAW*

The poor law tradition also speaks to the issue of relative responsibility. This legal tradition originated with the Elizabethan Poor Law of 1601.[16] The Elizabethan Poor Law was adopted by the American colonies and later incorporated into many state statutes dealing with the care and maintenance of indigent persons. For the most part, these laws have now been substantially modified or repealed, but their legacy remains.

One of the more important legacies of the poor law tradition is the relative responsibility statute.[17,18] The purpose of the relative responsibility statute is to shift, from the public to a number of different relatives, the responsibility for supporting the poor. The distinguishing feature of these statutes is that it extends the obligations under family law to relatives outside the nuclear family—grandparents, grandchildren[19] and, in some instances, brothers and sisters.[20] Some states have specified the order in which relatives become liable; most have not.[21]

The imposition of support obligations on relatives outside the nuclear family runs counter to the prevailing views of family structure. In American society, the nuclear family is accepted as the unit within which support obligations prevail. When children reach the age of majority and begin families of their own, moral obligation to provide support generally cease except that many adult children feel they have a moral obligation to support their aging parents. Legal requirements to support adult children or even grand-children are usually not reinforced by a corresponding sense of moral obligation.

The unfortunate aspect of the relative responsibility statute is that legal liability is usually imposed on relatives who are least able to support their kin. Poor persons often have poor relatives.[22]

Relative responsibility requirements have usually been applied to two areas of social welfare policy: (1) income maintenance, and (2) institutional care. A review of the statutes and litigation in both areas can be instructive with respect to the issue of rela-tive responsibility in home care.

## *INCOME MAINTENANCE*

Most relative responsibility litigation has involved the liability of adult children to contribute to the maintenance of their aging parents.[23] States generally have made adult children legally liable for their elders but this liability has not always been imposed in a consistent manner. Adult children who provide direct financial support to their parents are exempt from further legal action and parents are then considered ineligible for public assistance bene-fits.[24] However, an adult child's offer to provide direct support does not exempt him or her from reimbursing the state for the parent's income benefits even though the parent refused the of-fer.[25] In other words, legal liability does not necessarily stop once an offer to support a parent has been made.

Beginning in 1974, the federal government replaced the Old Age Assistance (OAA) program with the Supplemental Security Income (SSI) program.[26] One effect of this change was to shift more of the administration of income support payments for the aged from the state government to the federal government. Under the OAA program, states had considerably more discretion in es-tablishing eligibility criteria and in requiring relatives to support their older kin. There is no relative responsibility clause in the federal statute authorizing the SSI program. Because some states do supplement the federal SSI payment, it is not entirely clear whether the state relative responsibility provisions have survived the federal takeover of the income assistance programs for older persons.[27]

A second hotly contested relative responsibility issue is the responsibility of stepparents in households receiving financial support under the Aid to Families with Dependent Children (AFDC) program. The issue simply stated is whether stepparents are legally liable to support their stepchildren. This issue was put to rest by the U.S. Supreme Court in 1972 in the Boucher case.[28,29] Donna Boucher, a Massachusetts resident, faced a reduction in her AFDC grant when she remarried. The shelter portion of her grant was eliminated on the assumption that this part of her children's needs would be paid by the stepfather. The court ruled that the stepfather was not legally liable for the care of his stepchildren and that the AFDC family, therefore, survives the remarriage of the mother.

## INSTITUTIONAL CARE

Many states have also imposed financial liabilities on relatives for the cost of maintaining a person in a state institution, especially in institutions for persons with mental disabilities.[30] Some states specify the order in which relatives become liable; others do not. When the order of liability is not specified, the state agency enforcing the liability can choose to sue *any* of the liable relatives.[31] The only recourse for a defendant found liable is to plead with other legally liable relatives to contribute their support or to take independent legal action against them—a state of affairs that does little for family harmony.

Two cases are particularly noteworthy here. The first is the Kirchner case.[32] The California Department of Mental Hygiene charged the estate of Mrs. Kirchner for the cost of caring for her mother in a state institution. The Kirchner estate rejected the state's claim arguing, in part, that Mrs. Kirchner was not legally liable and that her mother had substantial cash resources of her own. The Department of Mental Hygiene argued that state law specifically mentions children as one of several relatives liable for the care of a person in a state institution. The department also argued that whether a patient has resources of his/her own was completely immaterial.

The California Supreme Court ruled that the Kirchner estate was not liable on equal protection grounds thus injecting a constitutional argument into the relative responsibility issue.[33] The court reasoned that because the purpose of state care was to protect both society and the confined person, the assignment of cost to one class of persons, i.e., relatives, violated the equal protection clause. The court noted that patients were exempted from paying for their care especially if it reduced their assets to a point where they would become a community burden once the patient was discharged to the community. To exempt patients, but not relatives—who might also be "denuded" of their assets—constituted an unequal protection of the laws.

However, the constitutional argument has not been shared by other state courts as in the second case—the Coty case which came before the Illinois Supreme Court a few years later.[34] The Illinois attorney general had taken action to collect from Louis Coty for the care provided by the Illinois Department of Mental Health to his mentally retarded son. The defendant argued that his liability to pay for his son's care was a violation of the equal protection clause of the federal constitution, since only one segment of society—the parents of a mentally retarded child—was being held liable. The Illinois Supreme Court acknowledged the California court's decision in the Kirchner case but rejected the constitutional argument and instead upheld the lower court's decision making Mr. Coty financially liable for his son's care.

## IMPLICATIONS AND CONCLUSIONS

What are the implications of these statutes and court decisions with respect to the liability of relatives in providing home care to a disabled person? While the courts have not spoken directly to the responsibility of relatives in providing home care, we can discern certain assumptions or conclusions that have guided the courts in their decision making. Moreover, these assumptions or conclusions, in one way or another, have also influenced agency policy in administering home care programs.

Our discussion thus far can be reduced to a number of key propositions outlining the parameters of relative responsibility:

—Husbands and fathers are legally liable to support their wives and children.
—Wives and mothers are not always financially liable but according to common law tradition are expected to provide in-kind support such as housekeeping and caring of children.
—Mothers are financially liable for the support of their children if the father fails or refuses to provide support.
—Stepparents are generally not legally liable to support their stepchild(ren).

—Support obligations within the nuclear family are enforceable under the doctrine of necessaries or by criminal penalties.
—An adult child can be made legally liable in some states to support an aged parent but the enforcement of this liability varies from state to state.
—Legal liability of relatives outside the nuclear family is usually specified for certain benefits or services such as income maintenance or institutional care. No liability is imposed outside the nuclear family for home care.
—While relative responsibility requirements have been challenged on constitutional grounds, most relative responsibility statutes have survived constitutional challenges.

We may conclude that whatever legal liability may exist for home care, it is mainly limited to the nuclear family. However, existing support obligations within the nuclear family do not preclude the state from supplementing those obligations with its own services. Existing relative responsibility requirements within the nuclear family merely gives the state a legal basis for withholding services (such as home care) if it so chooses.

To have real force, a legal obligation must be backed by a society's sense of moral obligation. In our society where the extended family is becoming more a thing of the past, the imposition of legal liability on relatives outside the nuclear family is fast diminishing. Moreover, the ability to enforce such requirements weakens as the financing and administration of public social programs shifts from governments that are local in scope to one that is national in scope. Finally, the changing roles of men and women in our society are causing a serious reevaluation of support obligations within the nuclear family.

While the concept of relative responsibility is rapidly weakening, it still has a strong residual effect on the formation of social policy. It is generally assumed that if another relative is living with a disabled person, the relative not only will provide the needed care, but ought to provide that care. Only recently have nonfamily members been providing in-home services to disabled persons on any significant scale. To date, the financial liability for such services has been limited to some measure of the family's ability to pay.

In the last couple of years there has been considerable discussion about "the family" and how it has been eroded not only by exogenous social and economic factors but also by the effects of public policy itself. The argument is that much of our public policy is anti-family. While the discussion on this topic is often vague and gimmicky, we can expect a new national awareness that will result in government action to supplement the support functions within the nuclear family.

## REFERENCES

1. There have been, however, a few instances of Federal legislation that have defined specific aspects of relative responsibility. For example, the 1965 amendments to the Social Security Act limited family responsibility to husband-wife and parent-minor child relationships.

2. For example, see Manby v. Scott, 1 Lev. 4, 86 Eng.Rep 781 (1659); Lungworthy v. Hockmore, 1 Ld. Raym. 444, 91 Eng.Rep. 1195 (1698); Bolton v. Prentice, 2 Str. 1214, 93 Eng.Rep. 1136 (1745); Evans v. Evans, 1 Hagg Cons. 35, 161 Eng.Rep. 466 (1790); Harris v. Harris, 2 Hagg. Cons. 148, 161 Eng.Rep. 697 (1813); Watkyns v. Watkyns, 2 Atk. 96, 26 Eng.Rep. 460 (1740); Lasbrook v. Tyler, 1 Chan.Rep. 44, 21 Eng.Rep. 502 (1630); Williams v. Callow, 2 Vern. 752, 23 Eng.Rep. 1091 (1717); Angier v. Angier, Gilb. Ch. 152, 25 Eng. Rep. 107 (1718); Head v. Head, 3 Atk. 295, 26 Eng.Rep. 972 (1745); Child v. Hardyman, 2 Str. 875, 93 Eng.Rep. 909 (1731); McCutehen v. McGahay, 11 Johns. 281 (N.Y. 1814); Bromley, Family Law, 4th ed. (1971); 1 Blackstone Commentaries on the Laws of England, 442 (Cooley 3d ed. 1884); 2 Pollock and Maitland, History of English Law, 405 (1895); 2 Burns, Ecclesiastical Law, 447 (4th ed. 1781).

3. Articles on the duty of support include Paulsen. Support Rights and Duties Between Husband and Wife, 9 Vand.L.Rev. 709 (1956); Brown, The Duty of the Husband to Support the Wife, 18 Va.L.Rev. 823 (1932); Crozier, Marital Support, 15 B.U.L.Rev. 28 (1935); Sayre, A Reconsideration of a Husband's Duty to Support and a Wife's Duty to Render Services, 29 Va.L.Rev. 857 (1943); Support of the Wife: Statutory Rights and Remedies, 28 Bklyn.L.Rev. 108 (1961).

4. For example, see West's Ann.Civ.Code (Cal.) Sec. 155, which provides that husband and wife contract towards each other obligations of mutual respect, fidelity, and support, and C.G.S.A. (Conn.) Sec. 46-10. See also the Uniform Civil Liability for Support Act, 9 Uniform Laws Ann. 219 (1957) enacted in California, Maine, New Hampshire, and Utah. A table showing support obligations in the various states may be found in 9C Uniform Laws Ann., 10.

5. Vernier listed twenty-three states having such statutes. III Vernier, American Family Laws, Sec. 160 (1935). See, e.g., A.R.S. (Ariz.) Sec. 25-215; West's Ann.Civ.Code (Cal.) Sec. 171; C.R.S. '63 (Colo.) 43-1-10; C.G.S.A. (Conn.) Sec. 46-10; S.H.A. (Ill.) ch. 68, Sec 15; I.C.A. (Iowa) Sec. 597.14; M.G.L.A. (Mass.) c. 209 Sec. 7; M.S.A. (Minn.) Sec. 519.05; V.A.M.S. (Mo.) Sec. 451.250; R.C.M. 1947 (Mont.) Sec. 36-109; R.R.S. (Neb.) Sec. 42-201; NDCC (No.Dak.) 14-07-08; ORS (Or.) 108.040; U.C.A. 1953 (Utah) 30-2-9; SDC (So.Dak.) 14.0206; RCWA (Wash.) 26.16.205; Code (W.Va.) 4752; W.S.1957 (Wyo.) 20-22. See Annot., Liability of Married Woman for Necessaries, 15, A.L.R. 833, 856 (1921).

6. Dreamer v. Oberlander, 122 Neb. 335, 240 N.W. 435 (1932), 18 VA.L. Rev. 680 (1932).

7. Bazeley v. Forder, 3 Q.B. 559, 565 (1968) (Dissenting opinion); 1 Blackstone, Commentaries on the Laws of England, 447 (Cooley 3rd ed. 1884).

8. Shelton v. Springett, 11 C.B. 452, 138 Eng.Rep. 549 (1851); 1 Blackstone, Commentaries on the Laws of England, 448 (Cooley 3rd ed. 1884).

9. E.g., West's Ann.Civ.Code (Cal.) Sec. 196; McKinney's Domestic Relations Law (N.Y.) 32; Merlino v. Merlino, 33 Misc 2 nd 462, 227 N.Y.S. 2d 262 (Sup. Ct. 1962).

10. See Cassas v. Cassas, 73 Wyo. 147, 276 P.2d 456 (1954). The rule in Iowa is different, the cases holding that both father and mother are equally responsible for the support of their child and may be required to contribute proportionally for that purpose, in accordance with their ability and circumstances. Picht v. Henry, 252 Iowa 559, 107 N.W. 2 d 441 (1961); Stillmunkes v. Stillmunkes, 245 Iowa 1082, 65 N.W. 2 d 366 (1954). State statutes and court decisions have only begun to consider the economic resources of the mother in establishing support requirements. For example, Plant v. Plant, 20 Ill. App. 3d 5, 312 N.E. 2d 847 (1974); Hursh v. Hursh, 26 Ill. App. 3d 947, 326 N.E. 2 dd 95 (1975). See Fisher and Saxe, Family Support Obligations: The Equal Protection Problem, 46 N.Y.B.J. 441 (1974); Conti, Child Support: His, Her, or Their Responsibility? 25 DePaul 2 Rev. 707 (1976).

11. Jordan Marsh Co. v Cohen, 242 Mass, 245, 136 N.E. 350 (1922); DeBrauwere v. DeBrauwere, 203 N.Y. 460, 96 N.E. 722 (1911); Grishaver v. Grishaver, 225 N.Y.S. 2d 924 (Sup.Ct. 1961); Daggett v. Neiman-Marcus, 348 S.W. 2d 796 (Tex.Civ.App 1961); Kerner v. Eastern Dispensary and Casualty Hospital 210 Md. 375, 123 A 2d 333 (1956); Mihalcoe v. Holub, 130 Va. 425, 107 S.E. 704 (1921); Feiner v. Boynton, 73 N.J. Law 136, 62 A 420 (1905); Mihalcoe v. Holub, 130 Va. 425, 107 S.E. 704 (1921); Greenspan v. Slate, 12 N.J. 426, 97 A. 2d 390 (1953) held that medical services furnished to a child were necessaries. Clark v. Tenneson, 146 Wis. 65, 130 N.W. 895 (1911); Read v. Read, 119 Colo. 278, 202 P2d 953 (1949, Price v. Perkins, 242 Md. 501, 219 A. 2d 557 (1966); Hayden v. Hayden, 326 Mass. 587, 96. N.E. 2d 136 (1950); Dravecko v. Richard, 267 N.Y. 180, 196 N .E. 17 (1935); Haynes v. Haynes, 192 Tenn. 486, 241 S.W. 2d 540 (1951).

12. Clark cites the following statutes. Clark, Law of Domestic Relations, 200 (1968). Code (Ala.) Tit. 34. Sec. 90; AS (Alaska) 11.35.010; A.R.S. (Ariz.) Secs. 13-801, 13-802, 13-804; Ark.Stats. Secs. 41-204, 41-205; West's Ann.Penal Code (Cal.) Sec. 270a; C.R.S. '63 (Colo.) 43-1-1; C.G.S.A. (Conn.) Secs. 53-304, 53-306, 53-309; 13 Del.C.Ann. Sec. 502; D.C. Code 1961 (Dist. Col.) Sec. 22-903; F.S.A. (Fla.) Sec. 856.04; Code (Ga.) Secs. 74-9903; R.L.H. 1955 (Hawaii) Sec. 328-1; I.C. (Idaho) Sec. 18-401; S.H.A. (Ill.) ch. 68, Sec. 24; Burns' Ann.St. (Ind.) Sec. 10-1401; I.C.A. (Iowa) Sec. 731.1; K.S.A. (Kan.) 21-442 through 21-445; KRS (Ky.) 435.240; LSA-R.S. (La.) 14:74; 19 M.R.S.A. (Me.) Sec. 481; Code 1957 (Md.) art. 27, Secs. 88, 96, 97; M.G.L.A. (Mass.) c. 273 Sec. 1; M.C.L.A. (Mich.) Sec. 750.161; M.S.A. (Minn.) Sec. 609.375; Code 1942 (Miss.) Sec. 2050 (children only); V.A.M.S. (Mo.) Secs. 559.353, 559.356; R.C.M. (Mont.) Secs. 94-301, 94-304; R.R.S. 1943 (Neb.) Secs. 28-446, 28-446. 01, 28-447, 28-449, 28-449.01; N.R.S. (Nev.) 201.020, 201.040, 201-050; R.S.A. (N.H.) 460-23; N.J.S.A. 2A:100-1, 2A: 100-2, 2A:100-3, 2A:100-4; 1953 Comp. (N.M.) Secs. 40A-6-1, 40A-6-2; McKinney's Code Criminal Procedure (N.Y.) 899,901; McKinney's Penal Law (N.Y.) Sec. 260.05; G.S. (N.C.) Secs 14-322 through 14-325.1; NDCC (No. Dak.) 14-07-15, 14-07-16; R.C. (Ohio) Secs. 3113.01, 3113.99; 21 Okl.St.Ann. Secs. 851-853; ORS (Or.) 167.605; 18 P.S. (Pa.) Sec. 4733; Gen. Laws 1956 (R.I.) Sec. 11-2-1; Code 1962 (S.C.) Secs. 20-303, 20-304; SDC (So.Dak.) 13.3201-13.3203; T.C.A. (Tenn.) Secs. 39-201 to 39-210; Vernon's Ann.P.C. (Tex.) arts 602-605; U.C.A.1953 (Utah) 76-15-1, 76-15-2; 15 V.S.A. (Vt.) Secs. 202-207; Code 1950 (Va.) Sec. 20-61; RCWA (Wash.) 26.20.030; Code (W.Va.) 4777-4781; W.S.A. (Wis.) 52.05, 52.055; W.S. 1957 (Wyo.) Sec. 20-71. Annot. 14 A.L.R. 1482, 1485 (1921). For a discussion of all aspects of criminal non-support see Jones. The Problem of Family Support: Criminal Sanctions for the Enforcement of Support, 38 N.C.L. Rev. 1 (1959).

13. Criminal sanctions are often counterproductive since there can be no support from the father should he be incarcerated. The court will often suspend the sentence on the condition that the father provide a specific amount of support for his children.

14. E.g., Code 1950 (Va.) Secs. 20-61.

15. E.g., S.H.A. (Ill.) Ch. 68, Secs. 24.

16. 43 Eliz. 1, ch. 2, Sec. 7 (1601), provided that the father, grandfather, mother, grandmother, and children of every poor, old, blind, lame, and impotent person or other poor person not able to work, being of sufficient ability shall, at their own charges, relieve and maintain every such poor person according to the rate assessed by the justice of the peace.

17. Some of the leading articles on this subject include: Mandelker, Family Responsibility Under the American Poor Laws, 54 Mich.1.Rev. 497, 607 (1956); ten Broek, California's Dual System of Family Law: Its Origin, Development and Present Status, 16 Stan.L.Rev. 257, 900 (1964), and 17 Stan.L.Rev. 614 (1965); Lewis and Levy, Family Law and Welfare Policies: The Case for "Dual Systems," 54 Cal.L.Rev. 748 (1966); Weyrauch, Dual Systems of Family Law: A Comment, 54 Cal.L.Rev. 781 (1966); Reich, Individual Rights and Social Welfare: The Emerging Legal Issues, 74 Yale L.J. 1245 (1965); Polier, Problems Involving Family and Child, 66 Colum.L.Rev. 305 (1966); Tulley, Family Responsibility Laws: An Unwise and Unconstitutional Imposition, 5 Fam. L.Q. 32 (1971).

18. Code (Ala.) Tit. 44 Sec. 8; AS (Alaska) 47.25.230; Ark.Stats. Sec. 59-115; West's Ann.Civ.Code (Cal.) Secs. 206, 241-254; C.R.S. '63 (Colo) 36-10-7; C.G.S. A. (Conn.) Sec. 17-320; 13 Del.C.Ann. Sec. 501; Code (Ga.) Sec. 23-2302; R.L.H. 1955 (Hawaii) Sec. 330-22; I.C. (Idaho) Sec. 32-1002; S.H.A. (Ill.) ch. 68, Sec. 52; Burns' Ann.St. (Ind.) Sec. 3-3001; I.C.A. (Iowa) Sec. 252.2; KRS (Ky.) 405.080; LSA-R.S. (La.) tit. 13 Sec. 4731; 22 M.R.S.A. (Me.) Sec. 4467; M.G.L.A. (Mass.) c. 117 Sec. 6; M.C.L.A. (Mich.) Sec. 401.2; M.S.A. (Minn.) Sec. 261.01; Code 1942 (Miss.) Sec. 7357; R.C.M. 1947 (Mont.) Sec. 71-233; R.R.S.1943 (Neb.) Sec. 6S-101; R.S.A. (N.H.) Sec. 167.2; N.J.S.A. 44:1-140; 1953 Comp. (N.M.) Secs. 13-1-27.1. 13-1-45; McKinney's Domestic Relations Law (N.Y.) 32: NDCC (No.Dak.) 50-01-19; 10 Okl.St.Ann. Sec. 12; ORS (Or.) 167.635, 416.010, 416.060; 62 P.S. (Pa.) Sec. 1973; Gen.Laws 1956 (R.I.) Sec. 40-8-13; Code 1952 (S.C.) Secs. 15-1228, 15-1229, 15-1230, 15-1231; SDC (S.D.) 14.0312; U.C.A. 1953 (Utah) 17-14-1, 17-14-2; 33 V.S.A. (Vt.) Sec. 931; Code 1950 (Va.) Sec. 20-88; Code (W.Va.) Sec. 626 (150); W.S.A. (Wis.) Sec.52.01.

19. E.g., Alabama, Alaska, Colorado, Iowa, Maine, Minnesota, Mississippi, Nebraska, New Jersey, Rhode Island, South Carolina, Utah, under statutes cited supra, note footnote #18. But grandparents of an illegitimate child are not held liable. State Board of Child Welfare v. P.G.F., 57 N.J.Super. 370, 154 A.2d 746 (1959).

20. E.g., Alabama (brother only), Alaska, Colorado, Illinois, Minnesota, Mississippi, Nebraska, Nevada, Utah, West Virginia, under statutes cited supra. note footnote #18. Stepfathers are made liable for support of their stepchildren by the statutes of California, New Hampshire, and South Carolina.

21. E.g., Alaska, Delaware, Illinois, Minnesota, Montana, Utah, and West Virginia, under statutes cited supra, note footnote #18.

22. One intent of relative responsibility laws is to spare the public purse. However, as some critics have pointed out, this intent is frustrated by the high cost of collection. See for example, Tulley, Family Responsibility Laws: An Unfair and Unconstitutional Imposition, 5 Fam.L.Q. 32 (1971).

23. Conant v. State et al., 197 Wash. 21, 84 lac. 2d 378 L (1938); Howlett v. State Social Security Commission, 347 Mo. 784 (1941); Manmouth Co. Welfare Bd. v. Coward, 206 A.2d 610 (1964); Re Commendatore's Estate, 255 N.Y.S. 2d 957 (1965); Mallatt v. Luin, 206 Or. 678, 294 P.2d 871 (1956); Carleson v. Superior Court, 100 Cal. Rpts. 635 (1972). See Tulley, Family Responsibility Laws: An Unwise and Unconstitutional Imposition, 5 Fam.L.Q. 32 (1971).

24. E.g., Howlett v. State Social Security Commission, 347 Mo. 784 (1941).

25. In Manmouth County Welfare Board v. Coward 206 A 2d 610 (1964) the court ruled that Coward's offer to support his aged mother did not relieve him of having to pay the county for his mother's Old Age Assistance.

26. 42 U.S.C.A. Sec. 1381 *et. Seq.* (1974), Pub. L. No. 93-603 Sec. 303 (a).

27. The 16 states that chose to administer their own supplemental payment (the state may elect to have the federal government administer the supplemental payment) are free to apply their filial support laws. Lopes, Filial Support and Family Solidarity 5 Pacific L.Q. 508 (1975).

28. Boucher v. Minter, 349 F. Supp. 1240 (1972).

29. See also Lewis v. Martin 397 U.S. 552, 90 S.Ct. 1282 (1970).

30. E.g., West's Ann.Welf. & Inst. Code (Cal.) Secs. 903 and 6650; C.R.S. '63 (Colo.) 43-3-1; D.C. Code 1961 (Dist. Col.) Sec. 21-586; Burns's Ann. St. (Ind.) Sec. 22-401 and 22-402; K.S.A. (Kan.) 59-2006; N.R.S. (Nev.) 428.070; Vernon's Ann. Civ. St. (Tex.) art. 3196a; RCWA (Wash.) Sec. 13.04.100.

31. Lister v. Sheridan, 33 Misc. 2d 650, 226 N.Y.S. 2d 323 (Sup.Ct. 1962); McManus v. Anonymous, 35 Misc. 2d 265, 229 N.Y.S. 2d 103 (Dist.Ct. 1962).

32. Department of Mental Hygiene v. Kirchner, 60 Cal. 2d, 716, 36 Cal. Rptr. 488, 388 P. 2d 720 (1964).

33. The first opinion did not indicate which constitution the California court was applying. When the case came to the Supreme Court of the United States, it was remanded on the ground that it could not say that the United States Constitution was the sole basis for the decision. On the remand the California Supreme Court held that it had been applying the California Constitution, although it would have reached the same result on the basis of the United States Constitution. Department of Mental Hygiene v. Kirchner, 62 Cal. 2d 586. 400 P. 2d 321 (1965).

34. Department of Mental Health v. Coty, 38 Ill. 2d 602, 232 N.E. 2d 686 (1967).

# Families, Care of the Handicapped, and Public Policy

Robert M. Moroney

## *INTRODUCTION*

Large numbers of Americans are convinced that significant changes in the family have occurred. The family is viewed as a social institution under attack, one that has been weakened over the preceding decades, one that is in danger of annihilation. This deterioration, in turn, is the reason why modern families are unable or unwilling to carry out those functions that have historically been their responsibility. It is further charged that those functions which include child care and the care of the handicapped and ill are being transferred to extra-familial institutions—the social welfare system. We hear complaints that parents are being shunted off to nursing homes or retirement homes by their adult children and handicapped children to institutions by their parents. More and more people, including elected officials, are arguing that government must find ways to restore the family to its earlier position of strength, to reverse the trend. To do so, it is suggested, would be in the best interest of society and the American family. Implicit in this position is the belief that families should care for their dependent members, especially the handicapped, and that families in the past were more caring and responsible.

This concern is not new. For example, the issue of family responsibility for the care of dependent persons, e.g., children, the handicapped, the elderly, has been the subject of continuous debate over the past three hundred and fifty years. Most social welfare programs have been developed on the premise that the family con-

This paper was presented at the Symposium on Family Policy, Florence Heller School, Brandeis University, Waltham, Massachusetts, November 7-8, 1978. It draws on research supported by the National Institute of Mental Health (NIMH-SM-77-0016) which was published in 1979 under the title *Families, Social Services and Social Policy: The Issue of Shared Responsibility*. Washington, D.C. DHEW, GPO. 1979.

stituted the first line of responsibility when individuals had their self-maintaining capacities impaired or threatened. It was further expected that families would support these persons until the situation became overwhelming and then, and only then, would society, either through the public or private sector, intervene.

This approach has been based on the principle that family life is and should be a private matter, an area that the State should not encroach upon. The family was and is viewed as the last sanctuary that individuals could retreat to, and as a fragile institution needed to be protected. The appropriate role of the State, then, was to develop policies that would protect and strengthen families. More often than not this has resulted in intervention only when absolutely necessary. "Necessary" involvement was, however, never clear and subject to various interpretations.

If this shifting of responsibility is taking place, if families today are increasingly giving up this caring function, and if the State is being looked upon as the primary source of social care for handicapped persons, such a trend has serious economic and social implications. How much social care can the State afford to provide? What form of society would we be moving toward?

For many people, there is little question about this shifting of responsibility. It exists. Policy-makers, planners, and administrators point to the increased demand for social services and the mushrooming of public and private expenditures for social welfare programs. Human service professionals who have direct contact with families, e.g., physicians, nurses, social workers, and therapists, conclude the same from their growing caseloads, especially the numbers of families who are seeking institutional care for their aged parents or handicapped children.

Some argue that this shift is related to a larger evolutionary process in which the nature of the family itself is changing. In its emerging form, characterized as more isolated than the extended family of the nineteenth and eighteenth centuries, the family as structured cannot function effectively as caregivers. Society, then, must respond by changing its perception of the caring function, and in doing so will of necessity expand the role of the Welfare State. This position begins with the notion of a weakened family system.

Others would argue that families may be less able or willing to provide care but see different causes. Family structure may be changing but the major reasons for families giving up their responsibility is related to how the Welfare State has been organized. Few services are available to support families. In fact, it is argued that services are designed to substitute for families.

A third position argues that in its evolution and expansion the Welfare State itself has adversely affected the family's willingness to provide social care. Intended or not, a growing Welfare State has weakened the family. In providing increased amounts of social welfare services, expectations have changed. Families are merely responding to policies that they interpret as encouragement or even pressure to transfer the caring function. In this sense, the State presents itself as a more effective institution.

From the above discussion a number of "facts" emerge. First, people are concerned about the health of the American family. They are convinced that it has been weakened and that this weakness has resulted in families divesting themselves of the care for their handicapped children and elderly parents. Second, people not only believe that this is happening, they are equally certain they know why it has happened and what should be done about it. Solutions range from expansion of the Welfare State, to restructuring the social welfare system, to dismantling the Welfare State through gradual retrenchment. Third, and most importantly, most of these beliefs, rationales, and recommendations are not based on a systematic analysis of relevant data. These positions are more often than not based on values or ideology and all too easily drift into an abstract debate about social ideals. Each group "knows" what is good, what should be done.

The remainder of this paper will examine the evidence with a view to clarifying this issue of family and State responsibility in the care of the handicapped. It is organized around three major topics. First, what do we know about the handicapped and families caring for handicapped persons? Are families giving up this function, as charged? If not, are they capable caregivers? Second, how does the Welfare State respond to the needs of the handicapped? What are our current policies? Under what conditions are services provided? The third and final section will attempt to present the underlying rationale behind our policies and their implications.

## THE HANDICAPPED AND FAMILY CARE

It is estimated that almost seven percent of the adult population has some impairment and as many as 2.5 percent are handicapped.

Table 1

Prevalence of Impairment and Handicap, 1970 (000)

| Age | Impairment | Very Severely Handicapped | Severely Handicapped | Appreciably Handicapped | Total Handicapped |
|---|---|---|---|---|---|
| 16-29 | 435 | 22 | 20 | 50 | 92 |
| 30-49 | 1,299 | 40 | 106 | 195 | 341 |
| 50-64 | 2,530 | 79 | 285 | 490 | 854 |
| 65-74 | 2,740 | 103 | 298 | 630 | 1,031 |
| 75 and Over | 2,855 | 260 | 405 | 574 | 1,239 |
| Total | 9,859 | 504 | 1,114 | 1,939 | 3,556 |
| Rates per/1000 | 67.99 | 3.47 | 7.68 | 13.37 | 24.52 |

Sources: Age specific rates from A. Harris. Handicapped and Impaired in Great Britain. Social Survey Division, OPCS, HMSO. 1971, pp. 5, 236; Social Indicators 1976. U.S. Department of Commerce: Washington, D.C. December 1977, p. 22.

Impairment and handicap can be defined in a number of ways and depending on the definition used, various estimates of incidence and prevalence can be derived. This analysis uses a functional definition rather than a diagnostic one. In the above table, impairment is defined as lacking part or all of a limb or having a defective organ which may be associated with difficulty in mobility, work, or self-care. Handicap is the disadvantage due to the loss or reduction of functional ability. Within this definition, not all impairments are handicaps. This approach is similar to the one used by the National Center for Health Statistics in its Health Interview Survey. Riley and Magi (1970), in their introduction to a review of these data, distinguish between impairment (anatomical and physiological abnormality which may or may not involve active pathology) and disability (the pattern of behavior that evolves in situations of long-term or continued impairments which are associated with functional limitations).

As mentioned above, almost seven percent of the U.S. population, or almost ten million people, have some impairment (Harris,

1971). Over 500,000 persons are very severely handicapped. This
grouping includes those who are mentally impaired or senile, unable to understand questions or give rational answers; or those who
are permanently bedfast; or those who are confined to a chair,
unable to get in and out without the aid of a person, unable to
feed themselves; or those who are doubly incontinent or cannot
be left alone since they might harm themselves. An additional
1,100,000 are severely handicapped. These include persons who
experience difficulty doing everything or find most things difficult and some impossible. The appreciably handicapped (about
2,000,000) can do a fair amount themselves but have difficulty
with some functions and require assistance.

Given current population projections, the impaired population
by the year 2000 will have increased by forty percent (an additional four million); the very severely handicapped by 200,000;
the severely handicapped by 450,000; and the appreciably handicapped by 800,000.

Neither impairment nor handicapping conditions are evenly distributed across the population. Sixty-four percent of all handicapped persons are elderly; seventy-two percent of them very seriously handicapped. Furthermore, elderly over seventy-four years

Table 2

Impairment and Handicap by Age (Rates per/1000)

| Age | Impaired | Very Severely Handicapped | Severely Handicapped | Appreciably Handicapped | Total Handicapped |
|---|---|---|---|---|---|
| 16-29 | 8.94 | 0.46 | 0.41 | 1.02 | 1.89 |
| 30-49 | 27.84 | 0.86 | 2.28 | 4.18 | 7.32 |
| 50-64 | 85.08 | 2.65 | 9.59 | 16.47 | 28.71 |
| 65-74 | 220.24 | 8.28 | 23.99 | 50.67 | 82.94 |
| 75 and Over | 372.60 | 33.91 | 52.92 | 74.90 | 161.73 |
| Total | 6 7.99 | 3.47 | 7.68 | 13.37 | 24.52 |

Sources:  Adapted from A. Harris.  Handicapped and Impaired in Great Britain.
Social Survey Division, OPCS, HMSO.  1971, pp. 5, 236.

of age are two and a half times more likely to be very severely
handicapped compared to those between sixty-five and seventy-four
years of age.

Data on children and youth are more difficult to come by. Riley
and Nagi (1970) state that two per one thousand under the age of
seventeen are handicapped. This seems a reasonable estimate given
the estimate of 1.9 per one thousand for those aged sixteen to
twenty-nine. Again, it should be emphasized that by definition,
handicapped is related to functional ability and not the presence of
an impairment.

Taking the rate reported by Riley and Nagi (two per one thousand under seventeen years of age), the total handicapped population is estimated at 3.7 million children and adults. This is a
significant number of people overall, a population that is at risk,
has a need for considerable services, and is potentially a high
user of the social welfare system. Not only that, but in light of
the discussion, it is a group that will make demands on families,
possibly heighten stress on family life, and at a minimum, force
families with handicapped members to function differently than
most families. Are families providing social care? Are families
transferring the caring function to other institutions?

Since 1950 slightly over one percent of the population has been
institutionalized. These institutions, moreover, include non-handicapped as well as handicapped. While there have been shifts in the
rates of institutionalization within categories of facilities, e.g.,
mental hospitals and facilities for the elderly, the overall rate has
been remarkably constant. Between 1950 and 1970 the institutional rate has dropped for each grouping below seventy, with the
largest decreases in the population under fifteen years of age.
Although the data in Table 4 do not present rates of institutionalization in the same age categories as the prevalence rates of
handicaps (Table 2), it is clear that in all age groupings, rates
of institutionalization are significantly lower than rates of handicapped persons.

Institutionalization, then, is not the norm. Most handicapped
persons, regardless of age, are living in the community. Some do
live in community facilities, e.g., shelters or small group homes;
others live by themselves *or* with families. It is this latter group
that is important for the purposes of this discussion. Since it is
impossible to deal with the handicapped in general (more often
than not the data do not exist), two groups of handicapped popu-

Table 3

Institutional Population - Rates per 1000 Population

|  | 1950 | 1960 | 1970 |
|---|---|---|---|
| Mental Hospitals | 4.06 | 3.43 | 2.13 |
| Mental Handicap | .89 | .95 | .99 |
| Homes for Aged/ Nursing Homes | 1.96 | 2.56 | 4.56 |
| TB/Chronic Disability | .50 | .35 | .08 |
| Homes for Neglected | .64 | .40 | .23 |
| Physical Handicap | .14 | .13 | .11 |
| Other | 2.17 | 2.48 | 2.40 |
| Total | 10.36 | 10.30 | 10.50 |

lations have been singled out for further analysis. A number of reasons can be offered to justify this decision. First, the size of these "at risk populations" and the pressures and problems faced by these families have serious implications for future resource allocations. Second, it can be argued that any shifts in the relationship between caregivers or changes in attitudes about who should provide social care will be first seen in these families. Over the past twenty-five years and especially since 1960, the State has made a commitment to these two groups, the elderly and the mentally retarded, and relative to other groups of dependents, they have been identified as groups to be given high priority in the development of social programs. Again, relative to other groups, there is now less stigma attached to aging and mental retardation. The former is a natural process, one which most individuals will experience, while the latter handicapping condition, especially severe mental retardation, is no longer viewed as the fault of the individual or family. In the terminology of the Poor Law, they are "worthy" of support. Given these factors, increased commitment of resources and decreased stigmatization, if there were a transfer of the caring responsibility from families to the social welfare system, it would likely be observed with these two groups of families.

Over the past twenty-five years, between five and six percent of the elderly population have been residents in institutions at the time of the decennial census. Most of these people are in nursing homes, homes for the aged, and mental hospitals. The data in Table 5 include these three rather than just nursing homes. While rates of institutionalization for nursing homes have increased significantly (from 19.6 per 1000 in 1950 to 45.6 per 1000 in 1970), this increase on face value is misleading. During the 1960s, many elderly patients in mental hospitals were transferred to nursing homes with the inception of Medicaid. These massive relocations were due in great part to financial reimbursements since the Federal government shared the cost of nursing home care while states bore most of the costs of mental hospital care.

These numbers, however, must be put in perspective. Over the past twenty-five years, between ninety-four and ninety-five percent of the elderly population have been living in non-institutional settings. Almost all elderly persons live in households, the majority in primary families.

A large number of the elderly are living with their children or

Table 4

Institutional Population, 1950-1970

Rates per 1000 by Age

| Age | 1950 | 1960 | 1970 | % Change 1950-1970 |
|---|---|---|---|---|
| Under 5 | 1.0 | 0.7 | 0.5 | -50 |
| 5-9 | 3.5 | 2.3 | 1.7 | -51 |
| 10-14 | 7.1 | 5.3 | 4.4 | -38 |
| 15-19 | 9.2 | 9.8 | 8.5 | - 8 |
| 20-59 | 10.3 | 9.9 | 7.8 | -24 |
| 60-64 | 16.3 | 15.2 | 11.6 | -29 |
| 65-69 | 17.8 | 17.7 | 16.7 | - 6 |
| 70-74 | 25.5 | 26.4 | 26.8 | + 5 |
| 75-79 } | 47.3 | 43.4 | 51.9 } | +49 |
| 80-84 | | 77.8 | 102.1 | |
| Over 84 | 94.1 | 126.3 | 179.8 | +91 |
| | | | | |
| Total | 10.4 | 10.3 | 10.5 | |

FAMILY HOME CARE

Table 5

Nursing Homes, Homes for the Aged, Mental Hospitals

(Rates per 1000)

| | 1950 | 1960 | 1970 |
|---|---|---|---|
| Males | | | |
| 65-69 | 17.71 | 16.27 | 14.88 |
| 70-74 | 23.72 | 22.41 | 22.00 |
| 75-79 | 34.94 | 34.36 | 37.96 |
| 80-84 | 51.89 | 58.36 | 70.49 |
| 85+ | 79.97 | 95.20 | 122.98 |
| Females | | | |
| 65-69 | 14.25 | 14.40 | 14.55 |
| 70-74 | 23.55 | 25.13 | 27.03 |
| 75-79 | 39.93 | 45.33 | 56.35 |
| 80-84 | 65.40 | 84.51 | 114.22 |
| 85+ | 97.71 | 136.47 | 200.15 |
| Total | | | |
| 65-69 | 15.70 | 15.28 | 14.69 |
| 70-74 | 23.64 | 23.87 | 24.83 |
| 75-79 | 37.30 | 40.45 | 48.86 |
| 80-84 | 59.39 | 73.72 | 97.45 |
| 85+ | 90.59 | 120.38 | 172.45 |

other relatives as their dependents. In 1970, this represented almost two and a half million elderly, of whom 1.8 million were
living with their adult children. Although this percentage has been
decreasing since 1950 (from twenty-one percent to twelve percent
in 1970), the absolute numbers have remained constant.

While these data might be used to support the thesis that families
are less willing to provide care, this conclusion is not warranted
since the age composition of the two groups is considerably dif-

ferent. In 1950, of those elderly living with their children or other relatives, forty-six percent were seventy-five years of age or older and seventy-one percent were women. By 1970, fifty-seven percent were in the older age category and seventy-eight percent were women. The latest data, 1976, show that sixty-two percent are the older aged and eighty percent are women. What seems to have happened is not that families are giving up the caring function for their parents who are handicapped (note the institutional rates over these same years), but that many of the elderly who are physically and mentally capable of caring for themselves are living alone or with just a spouse. Twenty-five years ago there was a housing shortage, especially housing for the elderly. Many elderly persons were forced to live with relatives. Today, those living as dependents are just that.

Families providing care to severely retarded children are different from those with frail elderly in a number of ways. Although the intensity of the stress and the nature of the demands are often the same, e.g., financial, physical, emotional, etc., the differences warrant a separate analysis. The aging process is perceived as normal, one which most people will experience. Furthermore, even though a number of elderly become dependent upon their children

Table 6

Living Status of Elderly 1950-1970 (Percentages)

|  | 1950 | 1960 | 1970 |
|---|---|---|---|
| Total | 12,244,380 | 16,197,834 | 20,091,825 |
| In Households | 94 | 95 | 94 |
| In Primary Families | 76 | 73 | 67 |
|   Head or Wife of Head | 69 | 56 | 54 |
|   Parent of Head | 15 | 12 | 9 |
|   Other Relative of Head | 6 | 6 | 3 |
| Living Alone | 18 | 23 | 27 |
| In Institutions/ Group Quarters | 6 | 5 | 6 |

or spend their last days in an institution, for most of their lives they are independent. Even the relatives providing care for the two and a half million elderly living in families as dependents know that this will end in a matter of years and they can pick up their lives after their parent dies. In most cases, also, these families have led normal lives before these demands were made.

Given the medical and technological advances of the past few decades, the severely mentally retarded child can be expected not only to survive childhood, but the majority will live an adult life. Parents are confronted with the possibility of providing care for the rest of their lives unless they decide to place the child in an institution. For these families, a "normal life" has to be redefined.

As argued earlier, an analysis of these two different but in other ways similar types of families should provide some insight into the kinds of social policies that might be developed. Additionally, their experiences should be generalizable to most families caring for handicapped members. Services that support families caring for a frail elderly parent or severely retarded child should not be too different in principle from those with, for example, a child with cystic fibrosis or a young adult who is quadraplegic. While the handicapped individual will require specialized services, the family is likely to need more generic services.

The prevalence of severe mental retardation (IQ 0-50) shown in Table 7 is drawn from the studies of Tizard (1974) and Kushlick (1964). The peak prevalence rate is estimated at 3.6 per 1000 persons aged fifteen to nineteen. This prevalence rate is probably close to the true prevalence rate for all age groups up to fifteen in so far as severe retardation is almost always present from birth or early infancy (Tizard, 1972). Given these rates, it can be estimated that there will be 561,000 severely retarded persons in the United States by 1980. Over 180,000 will be severely retarded children.

The projections for the next twenty years are based on extremely conservative assumptions. They begin with the position that the prevalence among children is not increasing substantially, and that the possibilities of preventing severe retardation are limited, given current knowledge. The projections further assume that the ratio of children to adults will remain the same, 1:2, although, as many more severely retarded children now are surviving to adult life, the number of adult retardates is increasing. Therefore

Table 7

Estimated Prevalence of Severe Mental Retardation (000's)

| Year | Under 15 | 15 and Over | Total |
|------|----------|-------------|-------|
| 1950 | 146 | 243 | 389 |
| 1960 | 200 | 271 | 471 |
| 1970 | 208 | 320 | 528 |
| 1980 | 184 | 377 | 561 |
| 1990 | 209 | 411 | 620 |
| 2000 | 211 | 449 | 660 |

NOTE: The rates used were: for the population under 15 years of age, 3.6 per 1000; for the population over 14, 2.2 per 1000 giving a total prevalence rate of 2.5 per 1000.

Sources: Population figures for 1950-2000 were derived from Social Indicators 1976. U.S. Department of Commerce, U.S. Government Printing Office, Washington, D.C., December 1977, p. 22.

the rate of 2.2 per 1000 for the population over fourteen years of age will possibly be higher. Regardless, the figures are useful, especially for the younger age group, and offer reasonable estimates for planning future services.

Severe retardation usually brings with it a range of physical disorders such as epilepsy, visual, hearing, and speech defects. Abramowicz and Richardson (1975) found that approximately one-half of all severely retarded persons have at least one additional handicap and that one in four have multiple associated handicaps. Their findings are supported by other studies (Conroy and Derr, 1971; Tizard and Grad, 1961). Table 8 gives estimates of type and degree of physical and behavior difficulties associated with severe retardation.

One in five of all severely retarded persons needs assistance in personal care functions; one in eight has severe behavioral problems, and one in fourteen is severely incontinent. With the exception of behavior problems, those under fifteen years of age are more likely to have associated handicaps. Children are twice as likely to be incontinent and need assistance in personal care functions and four times more likely to be non-ambulant. Eighty

Table 8

Incapacity Associated with Severe Mental Retardation

| Incapacity | Under 15 | 15 and Over | Total |
|---|---|---|---|
| Non-Ambulant | 24.06 | 6.23 | 11.45 |
| Behavior Difficulties Requiring Constant Supervision | 14.06 | 11.23 | 12.06 |
| Severely Incontinent | 12.55 | 5.20 | 7.34 |
| Needing Assistance to Feed, Wash and Dress | 28.33 | 15.49 | 19.25 |
| No Physical Handicap or Severe Behavior Difficulties | 21.00 | 61.85 | 49.90 |
| Total | 100.00 | 100.00 | 100.00 |

Source:  Adapted from Better Services for the Mentally Handicapped.
Cmnd 4683, HMSO, 1971, Table 1, p. 6.

percent of the severely mentally retarded children are likely to have a physical or behavior problem compared to forty percent of the severely retarded adults.

Based on the prevalence rate of 3.6 per 1000 for this age group, over 44,000 severely mentally retarded children are non-ambulant, 52,000 need assistance in feeding, washing, and dressing, 23,000 are severely incontinent, and almost 26,000 have severe behavioral problems.

Severe mental retardation is not, then, just a measurement of the intelligence level of an individual. For children it means that someone will have to provide care and supervision over and above what "normal" children require. This decision to maintain the child in the family setting seriously affects the family life of the other members. What are the institutional trends?

Eight of every ten severely retarded children and slightly more than two of every three of all ages are not in institutions, percentages that have remained fairly constant since 1950. Not all of these are being cared for by their families. A number may be in foster care, nursing homes, boarding homes, hostels, and other facilities. While it is impossible to determine the numbers involved, it is fair to estimate that, at least for children, most live

Table 9

Institutional and Non-Institutional Severely Mentally Retarded

|  | Estimated Number of Severely Mentally Retarded | Resident Population in Mental Retardation Institutions | Estimated Number of Severely Mentally Retarded in Institutions | % Not in Mental Retardation Institutions |
|---|---|---|---|---|
| 1950 |  |  |  |  |
| Under 15 | 146,000 | 25,845 | 23,260 | 84.07 |
| 15 and Over | 243,000 | 108,408 | 97,567 | 59.85 |
|  |  |  |  | (68.94) |
| 1960 |  |  |  |  |
| Under 15 | 200,000 | 46,269 | 41,642 | 79.18 |
| 15 and Over | 271,000 | 128,458 | 115,612 | 57.34 |
|  |  |  |  | (66.61) |
| 1970 |  |  |  |  |
| Under 15 | 208,000 | 48,141 | 43,327 | 79.17 |
| 15 and Over | 320,000 | 153,851 | 138,466 | 56.73 |
|  |  |  |  | (65.57) |

with their family if they are not institutional residents. This suggests that more than 165,000 severely retarded children will be living with their parents or other relatives in 1980.

Recent surveys of values and beliefs associated with family life, marriage, expectations, and roles of adults would argue against "family care." It is demanding, disruptive, and requires family members, especially the mother, to make major adjustments to family life. Although there are alternatives, e.g., nursing homes and institutions for the mentally retarded, most families apparently choose to provide care, often for long periods.

However, there have been slight shifts in institutional trends. While the data are inconclusive at this time and the long-term pattern still unknown, it is clear that once a placement is made, it usually means long-term care. There is also some evidence to suggest that families who are not provided support are less willing to take handicapped members back into their homes after an admission to an acute care facility (Morris, 1976; Beggs and Blekner, 1970; Lowther and Williams, 1966).

The literature documents the pressures and strains both sets of families (those caring for handicapped elderly and those caring for severely retarded children) are experiencing. Not all families are experiencing all of these stresses, but all of these families are "at risk" in that statistically they are more likely than families without handicapped members to have these problems. There are significant commonalities in the types of strains among both groups of families. In fact, they are probably common to families providing care to all of the physically handicapped. In turn, these pressures can be translated into the services that families could benefit from. They include:

—Additional financial costs (Newman, 1976; Sultz, 1972; Aldrich, 1971; Holt, 1958; Dunlap, 1976)
—Stigma (Schonell and Watts, 1956; Kershaw, 1965; Gottleib, 1975)
—Time consumed in personal care, e.g., feeding, washing, dressing (Shanas, 1968; Aldrich, 1971; Bayley, 1973)
—Difficulty with physical management, e.g., lifting, ambulation (Sainsbury and Grad, 1971; Shanas, 1968)
—Interruptions of family sleep (Bayley, 1973; Hewett, 1972)
—Social isolation, attitudes of neighbors and kin (Holt, 1958; Tizard and Grad, 1961)

—Limitations in recreational activities (Holt, 1958; Aldrich, 1971)
—Handling behavioral problems (Bayley, 1973; Justice, 1971; Younghusband, 1971)
—Difficulty in shopping and other normal household routines (Bayley, 1973; Younghusband, 1971)
—Limited prospects for the future (Bayley, 1973; Younghusband, 1971)

The family, then, is clearly not giving up the caring function. Large numbers of handicapped persons are living with and being cared for by their relatives—far more than are in institutions. The family has been instrumental in preventing or delaying long-term admissions to institutions, thus reducing a potentially heavy demand on social welfare services. Many families have provided what can only be described as a staggering amount of care and yet the evidence is that they want to do so. In this sense, the family has been a significant resource for handicapped persons and a resource for the social welfare system.

## SOCIAL POLICIES AND FAMILY CARE

Since the 1930s, the State has assumed that it has the responsibility to meet, either directly or indirectly, the income, employment, housing, and medical care needs of its citizens. In a sense, it guarantees their physical and social well-being. While this principle has been upheld by successive administrations, there has been little consensus as to which specific types of policies best serve the goal of promoting welfare or which interventions are more appropriate in achieving this goal. In fact, there has been a continuous and often bitter debate around these issues. The disagreement can be reduced to a number of fundamental questions. Should services be provided as a right or only made available to individuals and families when they demonstrate their inability, usually financial, to meet their basic needs? Should benefits be provided to the total population or restricted to specific target groups, usually defined as "at risk"? Should the State develop mechanisms to continuously improve and promote the quality of life or should it restrict its activity to guaranteeing some agreed upon minimum level of welfare, a floor below which no one is allowed to fall? Should it actively seek to prevent or minimize stressful situations both environmental and personal or should it react to problems and crises as they arise? On one level these questions are shaped by financial considerations; on another by disagreements on basic values. Arguments are offered that support the thesis that the country can afford only so much social welfare. Resources are limited and need to be given to those with the greatest need. Selective provision rather than universal coverage is viewed as more effective and less costly. In fact, selective provision is more likely to result in more services and higher levels of benefits for those truly in need and are not "wasted" on those individuals and families who can manage on their own. Finally, by introducing means testing or other criteria for eligibility determination, potentially excessive demand or utilization is minimized and the State will indirectly encourage individual initiative and responsibility. This position is countered with the argument that a residual approach, one that basically reacts to crises or problems after they have occurred, is short-sighted and that present economies might result in tremendous future demands. Furthermore, policies and services developed from this stance tend to stigmatize recipients, segregate them from the mainstream of life, and strengthen an already fragmented service delivery system.

The underlying issue is the relationship between families and the State. More specifically, it is concerned with the appropriateness of State intervention in family life. Under what conditions is intervention appropriate? For what purposes? In which areas of family life? What is appropriate for the family to carry out; what should they be required to do? What should be shared by both?

These questions are raised within a framework that builds on a number of key assumptions. The most basic is that the structure of the welfare state has been shaped by a number of beliefs concerning the responsibilities which families are expected to carry for the care of the socially dependent and a set of conditions under which this responsibility is to be shared or taken over by society. Admittedly, this framework assumes that both the family and the State have responsibility for the provision of care to dependent members. The legitimacy of this general proposition is rarely contested. Serious problems and disagreements emerge, however, when attempts are made to translate the idea of shared responsibility into specific social policies and programs, for then it becomes necessary to define which functions are appropriate to each. What does sharing mean in real terms and what is to be shared? What do families want the State to provide, and conversely, how does the State view the family?

There seems to have been agreement that society, through the State, had the right and responsibility to step in when individuals could no longer meet their own needs and did not have resources to fall back on. As early as the seventeenth century, the Poor Law made provision for widows with children through its outdoor relief policy. Children could be and were removed from their families and apprenticed if the State felt the family environment was not suitable. Today, this principle has been interpreted to cover the State's right to intervene in a family situation where a child has been or is in danger of being abused or neglected. The child is accepted by society as an individual with certain rights and one of these is protection from physical harm. Furthermore, few today would feel the State interferes with individual privacy when it removes an isolated elderly person to a nursing home when he or she is unable to meet basic survival needs. To the contrary, people are shocked and angry when they hear of an unattended elderly person starving or freezing to death. The emphasis in these situations is on the need to protect the individual who might harm himself, others, or be harmed. In these clear-cut cases, the State provides a substitute family in that it provides for some basic survival needs.

Over time the State has also assumed a degree of responsibility in less extreme situations where it is thought that families or individuals are unable to cope adequately. In practice, each generation appears to define what form of intervention is appropriate and under what conditions. This does not mean that each generation discards past policies and develops their own. The process has been incremental, characterized more by marginal adjustments than by radical change. Examples of these are the numerous income maintenance, food stamp, manpower, and educational programs. Intervention usually took place after a crisis or breakdown, whether individual or structural. While in the earlier period of the Poor Law, services were made available only as a last resort, forcing families to admit to pathology or "family bankruptcy," the current role of the State is still seen as marginal though not as repressive or personally demeaning. Legislation by and large still sees social welfare as a system concerned with a relatively small proportion of the population, a residual group unable or unwilling to meet their own needs. In general, then, the State has been reluctant to intervene if that intervention in any way was perceived to interfere with the family's rights and responsibilities for self-determination.

This residual approach, consistent with earlier social philosophies of laissez-faire and social Darwinism, is gradually becoming balanced with the belief that society, especially as represented by government, should assume more direct responsibility for assuring that basic social and economic needs be met. However, this evolution, incorporating many of the earlier Poor Law policies, has produced a number of uncertainties and the borderline between society's assuming increased responsibilities through its social welfare institutions and the family's retaining appropriate functions has become less clear. How has the State responded? Is there evidence of commitment? Are services such that they clearly emphasize supporting families or are they organized to take over the caring function when families are unable or unwilling to continue as caregivers? Who is the object of the policy or service—the individual or the family?

Expenditure levels show in relative terms the value a society places on social objectives. In this sense it can be interpreted as an indicator of the social welfare effort (Wilensky, 1975). Within this framework, the nation has made a commitment to the social well-being of its citizens. Expenditures have increased significantly over the past three decades whether measured by per capita expenditures (up 314 percent since 1950) or expenditures as a percent of the Gross National Product (up 1000 percent during this same period).

Within one Federal agency, the Department of Health, Education, and Welfare, a number of programs have been developed that in principle could be supportive to families with handicapped members. Thirteen of these are administered by Welfare, nine by the Office of Education, seven by the Social Security Administration, and two by the Public Health Service. These thirty-one programs were obligated at $102.7 billion in fiscal year 1976. Seventy-one percent of this total was accounted for by various income maintenance programs, twenty-five percent by programs paying for medical care services, and four percent for the provision of services. While this investment is significant, the distribution itself raises some questions. A fundamental issue in developing an improved support system for families caring for handicapped members lies in the dominance of the income approach. Federal policy has been

Table 10—Federal Programs Potentially Benefitting Families With Handicapped Members
(DHEW)

| Catalog Number | Agency | Title | Obligations Fiscal Year 1976 |
|---|---|---|---|
| | | **A. Specific Services** | |
| 13.427. | OE | Educationally Deprived Children/Handicapped | 96 M |
| 13.433. | OE | Follow Through | 59 M |
| 13.443. | OE | Handicapped, Research and Demonstration | 11 M |
| 13.444. | OE | Handicapped, Early Childhood Assistance | 22 M |
| 13.446. | OE | Handicapped, Media Services and Films | 16 M |
| 13.449. | OE | Handicapped, Pre-School and School Programs | 100 M |
| 13.450. | OE | Handicapped, Regional Resource Centers | 10 M |
| 13.520. | OE | Special Programs for Children with Learning Disabilities | 4 M |
| 13.568. | OE | Handicapped, Innovative Programs, Severely Handicapped | 3 M |
| 13.624. | OHD | Rehabilitation Services and Facilities | 720 M |
| 13.627. | OHD | Rehabilitation, Research and Demonstration | 24 M |
| 13.630. | OHD | Developmental Disabilities, Basic Support. | 32 M |
| 13.631. | OHD | Developmental Disabilities, Special Projects | 19 M |
| 13.635. | OHD | Special Programs, Aging, Nutrition | 125 M |
| 13.636. | OHD | Special Programs, Aging, Research and Development. | 6 M |
| Total. | | | 1,247 M |
| | | **B. Income Maintenance** | |
| 13.761. | SRS | Public Assistance-Maintenance | 5.9 B |
| 13.803. | SSA | Retirement Insurance | 45.1 B |
| 13.804. | SSA | Special Benefits for Those Over 71 | 185 M |
| 13.805. | SSA | Survivors Insurance. | 16.8 B |
| 13.806. | SSA | Special Benefits, Disabled Coal Miners | 961 M |
| 13.807. | SSA | Supplemental Security Income | 4.4 B |
| Total. | | | 73.3 B |
| | | **C. Medical Care--Financial** | |
| 13.800. | SSA | Medicare--Hospital Insurance | 12.2 B |
| 13.801. | SSA | Medicare--Supplementary Insurance. | 4.7 B |
| 13.714. | SRS | Medical Assistance Program. | 8.3 B |
| Total. | | | 25.2 B |
| | | **D. General Social Services** | |
| 13.600. | OHD | Headstart. | 462 M |
| 13.608. | OHD | Child Welfare, Research and Development. | 15 M |
| 13.754. | SRS | Public Assistance, Social Services | 16 M |
| 13.771. | SRS | Social Services, Low Income | 2.2 B |
| 13.707. | SRS | Child Welfare Services | 53 M |
| 13.211. | PHS | Crippled Children's Services | 77 M |
| 13.232. | PHS | Maternal and Child Health Services | 219 M |
| Total. | | | 3 B |
| Grand Total. | | | 102.7 B |

Source: Adapted from Family Impact Seminar. Toward An Inventory of Federal Programs with Direct Impact on Families.
George Washington University, February 1978. pp. 37 ff.

primarily an income policy, and while income supports are needed, their value may be lessened in the absence of a network of support services.

This general pattern raises a number of troublesome questions. The emphasis on income maintenance (71.4 percent) and the financing of medical care (24.5 percent) is based on the assumption that services are either less important or that individuals and families can obtain these services if they have the means to pay for them. This assumption, however, has not been borne out. In some instances there has been market failure; in others, the income support has not been adequate.

The income maintenance programs clearly support handicapped persons but are implicitly neutral toward the family. Their purpose is to offer protection against the loss of earnings resulting from retirement or disability so that the individual will not become indigent. The major exception is the Public Assistance Program which does have an emphasis on the family, but the existence of a handicapping condition is neither a part of eligibility determination, nor will it substantially affect the level of the benefit.

The second largest area of Federal expenditures is for medical care. Medicare, accounting for sixty-seven percent of these funds, primarily is used to pay for inpatient hospital care and services provided by physicians. Home health services accounted for only 1.3 percent of the total. Medicaid, on the other hand, can provide for a much broader range of medical care, including services in the home. However, less than one percent of the funds are used for these supportive services.

Approximately four percent of the total funds obligated were for the provision of social services. Of this $4.2 billion, seventy-one percent were for services to the general population, and the remainder was used specifically for handicapped persons.

Although considerably less is expended on services, even here there are major problems. As developed, most services are income related so that only those individuals or families with low income are eligible. While many families caring for handicapped members do receive and benefit from these services, more are ineligible. Again, this seems to assume that those whose income is too high to qualify have the means to obtain them. A final problem is that, with few exceptions, these benefits and services are provided to individuals and not to families.

Services and financial support are provided to handicapped persons, i.e., the elderly, the sick and disabled, the socially disadvantaged. The family is not the object of the policy or service. Little emphasis, if any, is given to supporting families caring for mentally retarded children or frail elderly parents. While these services and benefits may indirectly support these caregivers, they are not provided with this in mind and it is spurious to argue that if individuals living in families receive support, the entire family is supported. Such a belief may appear logical, but practice has shown otherwise. Overall, these policies have tended to ignore the family with a handicapped member, just as they ignore families in general.

## FAMILIES, SOCIAL POLICIES, SOCIAL SERVICES: A QUESTION OF FIT

A basic notion throughout this analysis is that the family can be defined as a social service. Although this concept is ambiguous and for some a term that demeans the family, it is a useful way to describe certain functions of the family. From a social policy perspective, it provides a framework for examining the relationship between families and the State and for identifying effective services. The essence of such policies and services is a commitment to the principle that families and other social institutions need to interact in providing support to handicapped persons.

Social services have come to be defined as those services designed to aid individuals and groups to meet their basic needs, to enhance social functioning, to develop their potential, and to promote general well-being. The starting point, then, is that families are a social service in that they, as well as the community, society, and the State, carry out these functions for family members. Furthermore, it is clear that families are providing more social care to handicapped members than are the health and welfare agencies. It is not argued that families are "better social services," that de facto they are better equipped to carry out these functions. Any statement such as this tends to bring sharp criticisms and examples where families are not capable or where individuals have been harmed by relatives. For example, few people are not aware of the rising numbers of reported child abuse or spouse battering instances. However, in general, families are functioning well in the care of children and other dependent family members. There is an American tendency to establish dichotomies, to argue that either families or the State should assume primary responsibility. For example, twenty-five years ago, professionals advised families with severely retarded children to place them in institutions. It was better for the child, it was better for the other children, it was better for the parents. Those parents who wanted to keep the child often found themselves under considerable pressure and were told that they had neither the skills, knowledge, or resources required to assist the child in reaching his or her potential. Many ambivalent parents were made to feel guilty if they resisted institutional care and they were led to believe that such a decision would not be in the best interest of the handicapped member in terms of his or her physical and social well-being. A second and equally convincing argument for institutionalization was that in providing care, intense strains are placed on the total family unit, creating problems for the other children or between parents. However, the pendulum recently seems to have swung to the opposite side. Professionals now seem to feel that community care, including family care, is superior to institutional care. Furthermore, it is extremely difficult, given current practices in the states, to institutionalize a young, severely retarded child. The current thinking among professionals is that institutional care is not in the best interests of the child or family as a whole, and much pressure is brought to bear on parents as was the case in the 1950s. While there have been exceptions to these polar positions, there has been a tendency to see solutions in either/or terms rather than to anticipate the value of diversity. It would seem that in some situations families can provide better care and in others, the State would be the more appropriate caregiver. Given this, there should be a range of policies and specific policies may have multiple purposes. Policies might then be located on a continuum whose end points are extreme forms of substitution (the State becoming the family for the individual) and total lack of State involvement in family life. The needs of families and individuals vary in time and over time, and ideally the State would respond to those variations with policies that support families when they need support and substitute for families when they are incapable of meeting the needs of their members. Even this postulation is incomplete since it suggests a progression from no services to supportive services to substitute services, the last only when the family breaks down. In many cases a family may need some other social institution to temporarily assume the total caring function of a child or a frail elderly parent but would reassume primary responsibility after the crisis has been dealt with. From this point of view, both functions (support and substitution) are necessary and neither can be offered as more important or desirable than the other.

If these premises are accepted, it becomes critical that current policies be evaluated and future policies developed within a framework where the family is identified as a social service interacting with other social institutions. The overriding question thus becomes: "What is the most desirable, effective, and feasible division of responsibility between the family and extra-familial institutions in meeting the needs of individuals and in what ways can these institutions relate to each other to maximize benefits?" As raised, the question emerges from certain biases. It presupposes the value of a relationship based on bilateral exchanges. It argues that neither institution is capable by itself. The data presented in this paper suggest that such an exchange based on the notion of shared responsibility does not exist. A number of reasons were offered to explain why this has happened. Two are critical and must be dealt with directly. The first is that, whereas families exist, they tend to be deemphasized or ignored when policies are formulated. The focus is primarily on individuals. The second reason is as complex. Whereas the notion that interference in family life is not sound, non-interference has come to be equated with non-intervention. Given this, services exist to take over family functions, but few are available to support families.

The case can be made that a caring society must involve some sense of shared responsibility. The essence of sharing begins with a recognition of the contribution that families are making. It requires also moving from a unilateral relationship to one based on exchange. If anything, families should be supported by a caring society if that society is concerned with its future.

## REFERENCES

Aldrich, F., et al. (1971). "The Mental Retardation Service Delivery System: A Survey of Mental Retardation Service Usage and Needs Among Families with Retarded Children in Selected Areas of Washington State." *Research Report*. Vol. 3. Olympia, Wash.: Office of Research.

Bagley, M. (1973). *Mental Handicap and Community Care*. London: Routledge and Kegan Paul.

Beggs, H., and Bleckner, M. (1970). "Home Aide Services and the Aged: A Controlled Study." Cleveland, Ohio: The Benjamin Rose Institute.

Conroy, J. and Derr, K. (1971). *Survey and Analysis of the Habitation and Rehabilita-*

*tion Status of the Mentally Retarded with Associated Handicapping Conditions.* Washington, D.C., Department of Health, Education and Welfare.

Dunlap, W. (1976). "Services for Families of the Developmentally Disabled." *Social Work.* Vol. 21. pp. 220-223.

Gottlieb, J. (1975). "Public, Peer and Professional Attitudes Toward Mentally Retarded Persons." *The Mentally Retarded and Society: A Social Science Perspective.* M. Begab and S. Richardson, Editors. Baltimore: University Park Press.

Harris, A. (1971). *Handicapped and Impaired in Great Britain.* London: OPCS, Social Survey Division. Her Majesty's Stationery Office.

Hewett, S. (1972). *The Family and the Handicapped Child.* London: Allen and Unwin.

Holt, K. (1958). "The Home Care of the Severely Retarded Child." *Pediatrics.* Vol. 22. pp. 746-755.

Justice, R., et al. (1971). "Foster Family Care for the Retarded: Management Concerns of the Caretaker." *Mental Retardation.* Vol. 9. pp. 12-15.

Kershaw, J. (1965). The Handicapped Child and His Family." *Public Health.* Vol. 80. pp. 18-26.

Kushlick, A. (1964). The Presence of Recognized Mental Subnormality of IQ Under 50 Among Children in the South of England with Reference to the Demand for Places for Residential Care." *Proceedings of the International Copenhagen Congress on the Scientific Study of Mental Retardation.*

Lowther, C., and I. Williamson. (1966). "Old People and Their Relatives." *The Lancet.* December 31.

Morris, R., et al. (1976). "Community Based Maintenance Care for the Long-Term Patient." Waltham, Mass: Levinson Policy Institute, Brandeis University.

Newman, S. (1976). *Housing Adjustments of Older People.* Ann Arbor: Institute for Social Research, University of Michigan.

Riley, L., and S. Nagi, (1970). *Disability in the United States: A Compendium of Data on Prevalence and Programs.* Columbus, Ohio: Ohio State University.

Sainsbury, P., and J. Grad de Alarcon. (1971). "The Psychiatrist and the Geriatric Patient: The Effects of Community Care on the Family of the Geriatric Patient." *Journal of Geriatric Psychiatry.* Vol. 4. pp. 23-41.

Schonell, F. and B. Watts. (1956). "A First Survey of the Effects of a Subnormal Child on the FAmily Unit." *American Journal of Mental Deficiency.* Vol. 61. pp. 210-219.

Shanas, E., et al. (1968). *Old People in Three Industrial Societies.* New York: Atherton Press.

Sultz, H., et al. (1972). *Long-Term Childhood Illness.* Pittsburgh: University of Pittsburgh Press.

Tizard, J. (1972). "Implications for Services of Recent Social Research in Mental Retardation?" *The Mentally Subnormal.* M. Adams and H. Lovejoy, Editors. London: Heinemann Medical Books. p. 272.

Tizard, J. (1974). "Epidemiology of Mental Retardation: Implications for Research on Malnutrition." *Early Malnutrition and Mental Development.* J. Cravioto, Editor. Uppsala: Almquist and Wiksell.

Tizard, J., and J. Grad. (1961). *The Mentally Handicapped and Their Families: A Social Survey.* Oxford: Oxford University Press.

Younghusband, E., et al. (1971). *Living With Handicap.* London: National Children's Bureau.

# Deinstitutionalization:
# Those Left Behind

Bonnie Brown Morell

The family is a critical factor in the deinstitutionalization of a retarded child. This is true whether deinstitutionalization is defined as the discharge of children from an institutional facility or as the prevention of their long-term residence in such a facility by providing them with alternate training or support in the community. In both instances, whether a child is deinstitutionalized depends heavily on the ability and willingness of his or her family to function as primary caretakers. This situation contrasts with that of most deinstitutionalized retarded adults, who are more likely to receive primary care in group homes, nursing homes, or sheltered apartments than within their own families.

However, in spite of the major role that families play in the deinstitutionalization of mentally retarded children, little progress has been made in implementing policies specifically designed to meet their needs. This lack of concern with the family at a policy level is in large part responsible for the continuing failure in the United States to decrease the number of retarded children receiving institutional care. Although social workers in the field of mental retardation have long been aware of the importance of the family, policies and programs relating to deinstitutionalization have focused primarily on the retarded individual.

This article will discuss the prevalence of substantial mental retardation among children in this country. A relatively low rate of deinstitutionalization among such children will be documented and will be contrasted with the greater progress that has been made in the deinstitutionalization of retarded adults. In addition, current spending patterns for direct services related to deinstitutionalization will be reviewed, and the discrepancy between these services and the needs of families with retarded children will be described. Finally, recommendations to increase the focus on families in policies and programs will be offered.

## OVERVIEW

The impact of deinstitutionalization is a major issue because 4 out of every 1,000 children between the ages of 5 and 19 in this country are affected by substantial retardation—that is, they have an IQ below 50.[1] It can be estimated on the basis of U.S. Census Bureau data that as of 1970, approximately 240,000 children in the United States were substantially retarded.[2] Of these children, 160,000 were being cared for in the community rather than in institutions; thus, two-thirds of the families with substantially retarded children in this country were caring for their child at home.[3] Because of the present emphasis on deinstitutionalization, parents with a child who is currently in an institution may be asked to consider having the child return home.

The burdens ordinarily involved in caring for a retarded child can frequently be increased for the family because substantial retardation is often found in conjunction with other serious impairments. Approximately one-half of the substantially retarded have at least one additional sensory or physical impairment. One-fourth have multiple handicaps in addition to being mentally retarded.[4] This frequently encountered combination of low intellectual functioning and related deficits presents many difficult medical and social problems. Because substantial retardation is a serious and permanent condition, families with retarded children cannot be expected to provide an adequate level of care at home unless they have access to specialized services for the child and general supportive social services for themselves. Although some progress has been made in the provision of care in the community to retarded adults, families with retarded children have not been receiving adequate help in maintaining these children at home. This is reflected in existing data on trends in the area of institutional care for children.

The provision of care in public institutions for the retarded rose more or less steadily for all age groups from 1950 to 1965.[5] In 1965, the number of persons in such public institutions was 97.6 per 100,000 population; by 1970, this rate had been lowered to

92.8 per 100,000 population.[6] A superficial examination of these figures indicates that deinstitutionalization has reduced the size of the population in institutions for the retarded. However, when data for all ages is combined in this way, the rate at which children and teenagers have been receiving institutional care is obscured.

As can be seen in Table 1, from 1965 to 1970, when the overall data indicate the beginning of successful deinstitutionalization, the rate at which children aged 5 to 9 received care in public institutions for the retarded rose from 85.1 to 108.0 per 100,000 population. In addition, although the rate at which children aged 10 to 14 received institutional care declined in 1970, 140.6 per 100,000 in this age range remained in institutions. In short, the decrease in the number of adults, not children, in institutions for the retarded has resulted in the prevalent claim that deinstitutionalization of the retarded is beginning to reduce the size of the institutionalized population.

When the characteristics of this population are examined, it can be seen that those currently residing in institutions are generally younger than previous populations because of an increase in the frequency with which those under 20 years of age receive institutional care. In 1970, 50.4 percent of the total population in institutions were under 20 years old, compared with 32.7 percent in 1950.[7] In addition, it has been estimated that a greater number of persons with low IQs reside in institutions than had previously been the case. In the mid-1960s, 82 percent of those institutionalized had an IQ under 50; by 1974, this figure had risen to 93 percent.[8]

TABLE 1. PERSONS RECEIVING CARE IN PUBLIC INSTITUTIONS FOR THE RETARDED, PER 100,000 POPULATION, 1950–70

| Year | Overall Rate of Institutionalization [a] | Age of Institutionalized Residents [b] | | | | | | |
|------|------|------|------|------|------|------|------|------|
| | | Under 5 | 5–9 | 10–14 | 15–19 | 20–24 | 25–34 | 35 and Over |
| 1950 | 85.3 | 11.9 | 53.7 | 124.9 | 181.6 | 151.6 | 118.8 | 64.1 |
| 1955 | 88.4 | 19.8 | 67.9 | 130.6 | 185.7 | 167.3 | 118.4 | 67.2 |
| 1960 | 91.9 | 17.1 | 77.2 | 139.8 | 197.9 | 177.1 | 123.6 | 66.2 |
| 1965 | 97.6 | 19.2 | 85.1 | 151.9 | 194.1 | 178.8 | 132.8 | 66.0 |
| 1970 | 92.8 | 41.9 | 108.0 | 140.6 | 161.1 | | 112.7 | 54.4 |

SOURCE: U.S. Department of Health, Education, and Welfare, *Mental Retardation Source Book* (Washington, D.C.: U.S. Government Printing Office, 1972), p. 24.

[a] Rate is defined as number of institutionalized persons per 100,000 population.

[b] Figures appearing for age groups are based on the number of institutionalized persons of a particular age per 100,000 population of the same age.

In addition, many young, severely handicapped children are staying in institutions for longer periods than in the past. For example, in 1960, 32 percent of the children aged 5 to 13 residing in institutions had been in the same facility for at least five years. In 1970, 42 percent of this group had been in the same facility for at least five years.[9] The most dramatic impact of deinstitutionalization can be seen at the other end of the spectrum: in 1960, 90 percent of the institutionalized population over 65 had been in the same facility for more than five years; by 1970, this figure had been reduced by one-third to 61 percent.[10]

Thus, as a result of deinstitutionalization, care for retarded adults has to some extent been shifted from the institution to the community. However, the needs of young, severely retarded children have not similarly been met within the community at large. This lack of progress appears to be attributable to the absence of adequate support for the families who generally would be expected to care for these children.

## *SPENDING AND SERVICES*

Given the large amount of money spent on programs relating to deinstitutionalization, an examination of current patterns of spending is necessary to understand the lack of progress made in reducing the rate at which retarded children receive institutional care. It is obvious that expenditures for many kinds of specialized services for the retarded have dramatically increased at the community level. For example, Maine spent $70,000 on community services in 1970, and $3 million plus another $2 million in local matching funds in 1976. Alabama spent $25,000 on community services in 1969, and $1.5 million in 1976. Similarly, expenditures in Arkansas in this area increased from $500,000 in 1971 to $2.1 million in 1974.[11] Nevertheless, much of this money has paid for programs that serve retarded individuals without considering the special needs of families with retarded children.

A large share of the budget for community services in many states has been devoted to the development of vocational training and employment opportunities for retarded adults. Sheltered workshops are one example of programs designed to provide such opportunities. They prepare adults for eventual employment in an unsheltered environment by molding the attitudes of participants, developing their physical capabilities, supplying them with vocational training, and providing them with assistance in obtaining suitable jobs. In 1968, 1,029 sheltered workshops were operating in this country.[12] By 1973, approximately 2,500 such workshops were in operation. In addition to sheltered workshops, 706 activity centers providing individuals opportunities for social development and preparation for work were operational in 1971.[13] These centers are designed to provide therapeutic activities for adults who are so severely impaired that they are unable to perform in a sheltered work environment.

Another major investment of funds appears to have taken place in the development of supervised group homes and sheltered apartments for the retarded. Although national data are not available, these community living arrangements usually seem to serve retarded adults who need only a moderate amount of supervision. In contrast, few options for short-term care in the community have been made available to substantially retarded children in need of constant care. Furthermore, the use of institutions as a short-term resource, a practice carried out in the United Kingdom, does not seem to be developing as rapidly in the United States.[14]

Another program for the retarded is the system of mental retardation clinics funded by the Maternal and Child Health Service. These clinics provide comprehensive evaluative, therapeutic, and follow-up services to children. Although 154 of these clinics were in existence in 1971, only about one-fourth of the substantially retarded children and their families in this country were served by them in 1970.[15]

Some services, however, have been instituted for retarded children in the community. One example of a community service for the retarded that is designed to serve children is the developmental day care center. By 1968 approximately 2,000 day facilities were in existence, many of which provided developmental day care services to retarded children.[16] Such facilities appear to be supportive of the family by helping children develop self-help skills and by giving parents some relief from caring for their child twenty-four hours a day.

A major change that has also lent support to families caring for retarded children at home has been the increase in access to public education for even the most severely handicapped children. Enrollment in special education classes for children with IQs below 50 increased dramatically from approximately 17,000 in 1958 to 148,000 in 1972-73.[17] This increase has been brought about primarily by federal legislation. The culmination of the trend to provide handicapped children access to education was the Education for All Handicapped Children Act (P.L. 94-142), which required that school systems provide a "free, appropriate public education" to all handicapped children in order to be eligible for federal funds. This law mandated that priority be given to developing educational opportunities for the most severely handicapped children and those children who had not previously been served. The commitment to handicapped children represented by this legislation is clearly a major boon to families attempting to keep their retarded child with them in the community. It may also be a factor in the decrease in institutional care received by those between 10 and 14 years of age, since the provision of educational and vocational training services in the community may be one alternative to such care for these youngsters.

As can be seen from this description of various community-based programs, the focus of service is primarily on the needs of the retarded individual regardless of age. Those programs that do serve children are based on policies concerned with the provision of a specific service to the retarded client rather than on the provision of assistance and support to the family. This fragmented approach is inherent in all specialized programs designed to serve individuals with specific disabilities. As valuable as these specialized services are, the failure to consider the needs of both the retarded child and his or her family may result in progress for the child at the expense of other family members.

## NEEDS OF FAMILIES

The financial pressure caused by providing care at home to a retarded child is a major stress for many families. A survey of families who were providing such care found that the most frequently cited adverse effect of maintaining a retarded child at home was the consequent impact on the family's budget.[18] Forty percent of the fathers and 44 percent of the mothers surveyed indicated a need for additional financial resources to maintain normal family functioning.

The extra medical expenses incurred in caring for a retarded child also place great financial pressure on most families. In examining data on the cost of medical care for children with chronic conditions including some forms of mental retardation, Sultz and his associates found that the burden presented by these costs was substantial.[19] In the year of the survey in which medical costs were highest, the mean out-of-pocket expenses sustained by the families studied for medical care for their handicapped child alone were equivalent to 6.6 percent of their mean gross income. This figure was much higher than for families in general, who were found to spend about 5.5 percent of their mean gross income on medical expenses for the entire family. The financial burden documented was found to be greatest for lower-middle-class families. In addition, 38 percent of the families surveyed suffered financial hardship due to the special medical needs of their handicapped child. Ten percent of these families were found to be spending almost one-third of their gross annual income on their child's medical care. Clearly, unless some changes in policy are made for the provision of medical care for retarded children to prevent their families from being financially overwhelmed, public institutional care will continue to be the most logical option available for these children.

The sources of financial aid that are currently available do not serve many families with retarded children. Some assistance is available through Medicaid to low-income families with retarded children having medical problems. However, because eligibility for such assistance is linked to level of income, many middle-income families are not receiving adequate help with their medical expenses.

Furthermore, although financial aid from several sources is available to help retarded individuals meet their living expenses, eligibility is often linked to the level of total family income and children are usually not the recipients of such aid. The Supplemental Security Income program replaced former public assistance programs to the blind and disabled in January 1974. By November of that year, however, only 65,000 children were receiving payments from this program, and data are unavailable regarding what percentage of these children were mentally retarded.[20]

Finally, some states such as North Carolina allow an income exemption of $2,000 for the care of a dependent with an IQ below 40 in determining the amount of state income tax due. Generally, however, little progress has been made in providing financial aid to the majority of families who are attempting to provide care at home to a substantially retarded child.

Moreover, financial problems are not the only difficulties faced

by the families of retarded children. The need for these families
to have preferential access to general social services becomes clear
when the everyday stresses imposed by the presence of a retarded
child in the home are considered. Many articles and surveys have
been published examining the effect on the family of caring for
such a child, and some of the aspects and activities of family life
found to be adversely affected are the maintenance of marital
stability, the completion of household chores, ease of obtaining
baby-sitters, and ability to partake of vacations and other recreational activities.[21]

The effect on normal siblings of a retarded child's presence in
the home has also been of major concern to both parents and
professionals.[22] In the past this concern often resulted in professionals recommending that the retarded child be institutionalized as
soon as possible to reduce the stress placed on the family. Currently, however, parents are often advised to keep their child at
home so that his or her life will be as normal as possible. Both
these positions fail to achieve a balanced focus that takes the
needs of the child and the rest of the family into account.

At present, all too often the needs of other family members
are considered only if they correspond to components of the specialized services provided to the retarded child. However, the success of deinstitutionalization is not only linked to providing specialized services for the child but also to increasing the family's access
to household help, child care, recreation, and job opportunities.

## POLICY RECOMMENDATIONS

Further progress in the deinstitutionalization of mentally retarded children is dependent on a shift in policy focus from the
child to the total family unit. This focus would have to concentrate
on providing families with relief from financial pressure, increased
access to general social services, and additional options for short-
term care.

As already indicated, the major need perceived by families was
for financial relief in order to maintain normal family functioning.
One policy designed to reduce financial stress, particularly for
middle-income families, would be to allow an additional exemption within the federal income tax structure for families caring
for a retarded child at home. Such a measure would be similar
to one already in effect at the state level in North Carolina and

would be a way to increase the money available to these families to meet the needs of all their members. The blind and those over 65 currently receive an extra exemption from paying federal tax. A similar measure enacted for the retarded would recognize that this group is also faced with unusual financial stress.

The pressure on families caused by the extraordinary medical needs of retarded children could also be relieved by establishing a system for the payment of medical expenses. Other groups in danger of being overwhelmed by medical costs, such as the elderly and those with kidney disease, have been provided with aid. Until major changes take place and this country's health care system provides medical care to all as a right, the families of the retarded should be protected against the high cost of care.

One measure that would increase access to general social services for families of retarded children would involve the adjustment of income eligibility levels for local social services provided by Title XX funds. The social stresses on middle-income families as well as on poor families are sufficiently great to justify providing them with preferential access to services that are designed to strengthen families as caretakers and reduce the need for the state to substitute for the family by providing care twenty-four hours a day in institutions. The recognition that families caring for a retarded child are potentially in great need of a wide variety of social services could be built into the criteria for means-tested services if the income eligibility level for these families was raised.

Another change in policy that would acknowledge the needs of the total family would be the coordination of services for all family members. This change could be effected by the development of a management system for services, and such a system could be set up as a separate program or as part of an existing agency already serving the retarded.

The establishment of a family-focused case management system would be particularly beneficial because the current pattern of service delivery involves many different agencies. Each agency offering specialized services is apt to be in contact with only a small percentage of families with retarded children, as is the case with the mental retardation clinics funded by the Maternal and Child Health Service. An effective management system would reduce the difficulties faced by families in obtaining both specialized services for the retarded and general social services. Personnel involved in such a system could work with parents in a periodic review of the needs of the whole family and assist them to obtain appropriate services. Help in the form of job training for a parent or recreational opportunities for normal siblings could in many instances be the decisive factor that enables a family to continue taking care of a retarded child.

An additional measure designed to lend support to families would be the development of a greater number of options in the area of short-term care for retarded children. This could be accomplished in several ways. Existing institutions could modify their admissions policies and reserve space that would be available on short notice to children to relieve their parents temporarily of the responsibility of providing care. A community-based alternative would be the allocation of public funds to pay for short-term foster care by persons trained to meet the exceptional needs of retarded children in their own communities. Still another alternative that would be especially supportive to retarded children and their families would be the provision of public funds to train and pay special caretakers to act temporarily as substitute parents in the family's own home. This last form of care would avoid the disruption of the retarded child's access to ongoing community services such as developmental day care or school.

## CONCLUSION

The development of the options just described would enable families to keep their retarded child at home if they wished to do so by ensuring them the possibility of temporary relief when the needs of other family members required the full attention of the family as a whole. The changes in policy outlined have been suggested because legislative precedents exist for them. That is, their implementation would only require the modification of current laws to acknowledge and reduce the stress on families caring for a retarded child at home. It seems likely that the cost of these changes to ease the pressure on families would be slight compared to the cost of providing institutional care for retarded children. It also seems less significant than the social cost sustained by families who are struggling to provide care unaided by appropriate support.

By increasing the money available to families for everyday expenses, providing them with protection against high medical costs, easing their access to general social services, and creating options for short-term care, the changes in policy proposed by the author would enhance their ability to keep the retarded child at home. If deinstitutionalization is to succeed without imposing excessive stress on the families of the retarded, future policies must take into account support for the family unit as well as specialized services for the retarded child.

## NOTES AND REFERENCES

1. Helen Abramowicz and Stephen Richardson, "Epidemiology of Severe Mental Retardation in Children: Community Studies," *American Journal of Mental Deficiency,* 80 (July 1975), pp. 18-39.
2. U.S. Bureau of the Census, *Census of Population: 1970* (Washington, D.C.: U.S. Government Printing Office, 1973).
3. U.S. Department of Health, Education, and Welfare, *Mental Retardation Source Book* (Washington, D.C.: U.S. Government Printing Office, 1972), p. 24.
4. Abramowicz and Richardson, op. cit.
5. Alfred Baumeister, "The American Residential Institution: Its History and Character," in Baumeister and Earl Butterfield, eds., *Residential Facilities for the Mentally Retarded* (Chicago: Aldine Publishing Co., 1970), pp. 1-28.
6. U.S. Department of Health, Education, and Welfare, op. cit.
7. Ibid.
8. Earl Butterfield, "Basic Facts about Public Residential Facilities for the Mentally Retarded," in Robert Kugel and Wolf Wolfensberger, eds., *Changing Patterns in Residential Services for the Mentally Retarded* (Washington, D.C.: U.S. Government Printing Office, 1969); and President's Committee on Mental Retardation, *Mental Retardation: The Known and The Unknown* (Washington, D.C.: U.S. Government Printing Office, 1975), p. 63.
9. U.S. Bureau of the Census, *Census of Population: 1960,* Vol. 2: *Inmates of Institutions* (Washington, D.C.: U.S. Government Printing Office, 1963), p. 39; and U.S. Bureau of the Census, *Census of Population: 1970,* Vol. 2: *Persons in Institutions and Other Group Quarters* (Washington, D.C.: U.S. Government Printing Office, 1973), p. 61.
10. Ibid.
11. Raymond Nathan, ed., *Mental Retardation: Trends in State Services* (Washington, D.C.: U.S. Government Printing Office, 1976).
12. President's Committee on Mental Retardation, op. cit.
13. Ibid.
14. Robert Moroney, *The Family and the State: Considerations for Social Policy* (London, England: Longman, 1976).
15. U.S. Department of Health, Education, and Welfare, op. cit., p. 75.
16. Ibid., p. 71.
17. For data relating to 1958, *see* Romaine Mackie, *Special Education in the United States: Statistics 1948-1966* (New York: Teachers College Press, 1969); for data relating to 1972-73, *see* Edward Klebe, *Key Facts on the Handicapped* (Washington, D.C.: U.S. Government Printing Office, 1975).
18. Robert Aldrich et al., *The Mental Retardation Service Delivery Project* (Olympia, Wa.: Washington State Department of Social and Health Services, 1971).
19. Harry Sultz et al., *Long-Term Childhood Illness* (Pittsburgh: University of Pittsburgh Press, 1972).
20. President's Committee on Mental Retardation, op. cit., p. 60.

21. For a current review, *see* J. Carr, "The Effect of the Severely Subnormal on Their Families," in Ann Clarke and Alan Clarke, eds., *Mental Deficiency: The Changing Outlook* (New York: Free Press, 1975), pp. 807-838; and Aldrich et al., op. cit.

22. *See* Frances Grossman, *Brothers and Sisters of Retarded Children* (Syracuse, N.Y.: Syracuse University Press, 1972).

# Policy Responses to Schizophrenia: Support for the Vulnerable Family

## Aileen Florita Hart

Considerable legislative, scholarly, and media descriptions of the family suggest significant weakening of family roles or family ties. Deterioration of the family as a viable social institution in turn, is credited with the increasing use of institutions for the vulnerable family member—the aged, the physically handicapped, and the mentally disabled person. Implicit, general criticism appears to be that government provides too much and the family too little for its vulnerable members.

Coupled with a global concern for the perceived diminishing obligation of the family has been a trend toward deinstitutionalization. Deinstitutionalization is, in effect, shifting the care site from institutions to community and family loci. If such a trend is evident, who cares and who pays for the care of persons suffering from schizophrenia? Which responsibilities and costs are public? Which are private? Which are borne by insurance companies? Which by the family? What have been the consequences of such decisions to the individual, to society as a whole, and especially to the family?

The family of a schizophrenic is caught in a complex web of ambiguity and ambivalence. One aspect of this web is the lack of clarity concerning the entity: schizophrenia. A myriad of unknown and confusing factors exists, about which much dissent can be found among experts; these factors affect both diagnosis and intervention. Moreover, the lack of clarity concerning what constitutes schizophrenia is exacerbated by contradictory theories and little definitive evidence concerning the role of the family as causal agent. Both biochemical and socioculture research findings have been presented with equal strength of conviction by adherents on either side.

A second aspect of ambiguity affecting the care of the schizophrenic is the lack of legal and cultural definition regarding the

*225*

role of the family. To what extent should the care of a schizo-phrenic person be the financial and emotional responsibility of the family? Is the family the orchestrator or coordinator of com-munity resources for its schizophrenic member? Or does that task belong to the community mental health facilities? What is the role of the family, and what is society's role vis-à-vis the schizophrenic?

The chronic and cyclical nature of schizophrenia, together with the spotty and clinically inadequate nature of available community benefits, comprises another aspect of ambiguity for the family. Outpatient care for schizophrenics and their families, as viewed through the lens of available services, falls far short of the high rhetoric of Community Mental Health Acts.

Discrepancy and tension exist between the rhetoric and opera-tional reality surrounding the care and protection of the schizo-phrenic and his or her family. In this article we will examine several of these tensions by addressing three interrelated issues:

1. Alternative definitions of schizophrenia.
2. The costs associated with schizophrenia and who bears those costs.
3. Types of living and care arrangements for schizophrenics and whether they are available in the community.

This paper will address the implications of these three inter-related issues for the family. Special attention will be given to existing social policies as well as to alternative policy options and their potential effect on the family. Effects upon the family will be considered according to how helpful, neutral, or harmful they are to the family. The implicit or explicit responsibility that rests with the family will also be highlighted. Finally, the policy supports that are available to the family will be considered, as will recommendations for how the public sector can better support the family of the schizophrenic.

## DEFINITION AND ITS CONSEQUENCES

Mental health specialists disagree on which criteria are most effective in both the diagnosis and definition of schizophrenia. These differences in definition, as we shall see, have a direct bearing on the extent of family responsibility for the schizophrenic. In fact, the nature, etiology, and preferred treatment of schizophrenia have been among the more difficult problems ever to face mental health professionals. Over the last fifteen years some progress has been made in the development of applicable, standardized patient evaluation procedures.[1] These begin to make it possible to test the reliability of various diagnostic systems regarding etiology, prognosis, and effective treatment. However, rates of agreement in diagnoses still vary from 37% to 80%.[2]

Estimates of the prevalence of schizophrenia suggest that two million people in the United States, or up to 1% of the population, suffer from this disorder. Data suggest that over one million families are burdened with at least one severely incapacitated member who will remain ill and dependent throughout his or her lifetime.

A major problem in arriving at reliable data regarding prevalence is that a wide range of symptoms are used to define the disorder. Symptoms of schizophrenia[3] include perceptual distortion which may include auditory hallucinations; altered motor behavior ranging from peculiar mannerisms to frenetic or purposeless activity; thought disturbances leading to bizarre speech, illogical thinking, or distorted concept formation; and paranoid delusions— expressed as either pervasive suspicion or fully developed and complex belief systems concerning improbable plots against the individual. These plots include interpreting institutionalization as the jailing of an innocent against his will.

Because of variations like these, the diagnosis is often accorded to anyone exhibiting serious behavioral disturbance, marked impropriety of behavior, or expression in words that do not have shared meaning.[4] The problem of diagnosis is replete throughout the literature reporting research on etiology.[5]

Dissent concerning the descriptive definition of schizophrenia is compounded by a conflict among theories of etiology. Some researchers concentrate upon elucidating the specific nature of genetic, biochemical disturbances. Others define schizophrenia not as a disease at all but rather as a set of personality characteristics. Descriptions of the empty, meaningless, and lonely quality of life experienced by a so-called schizophrenic person are of value in that they stress the human factor, but they cannot be understood in genetic or biochemical terms. Nor are they generalizable as diagnostic criteria. Similarly, descriptions of genetic disturbance do not inform environmental theories of symptomatology.

In essence, there appear to be at least three major ways of

viewing the disease that are not in harmony with one another. One is physical and biological. Studies reflecting this point of view tend to focus upon hereditary transmission.[6] These use sophisticated means of studying twins and observing children of schizophrenic parents raised in adoptive families. Proponents of the physical basis of schizophrenia conclude that at least forty percent of schizophrenic cases are attributable to genetic factors.[7]

A second belief about etiology is essentially psychodynamic and interactive. It is characterized by concepts of functional behavior and relationships; it does not stress experimental study. Originally, Freud described schizophrenia as a narcissistic disturbance of person-object relations.[8] Other researchers followed suit and similarly stressed pathological regression to earlier developmental stages.[9] Proponents of this view point to disturbed family communications and interactions as the likely origins of schizophrenia.[10]

The third belief concerning the etiology of schizophrenia is phenomenological. Its proponents believe that schizophrenia is a "catch-all" category to include people exhibiting the variety of symptoms described here.

The theoretical differences notwithstanding, schizophrenia yields a set of major problems for the family. Due to the cyclical and chronic nature of the illness, minimal functioning and self-care are often the result. This means that the family is often plagued with the burden of living arrangements, costs, and referral to treatment facilities as appropriate, in addition to all that is involved in day-to-day care. The extent of responsibility borne by the family depends upon the orientation (and the definition of schizophrenia) implicit in social policies and programs. For example, if schizophrenia is defined as a physiological condition, insurance benefits could be expected to cover the direct costs of the illness such as medical care as well as indirect costs such as living arrangements. Conversely, if schizophrenia is defined as an interpersonal state rather than a medical condition, greater clinical attention is likely to be paid to the family members as causal agents. In the first case, relatively little emotional support may be available to the family. In the second, overemphasis on the family's culpability may stand in the way of providing support.

## THE COSTS OF SCHIZOPHRENIA

The total cost of care for schizophrenia is estimated to be $4.2 billion per year.[11] Gunderson and Mosher assess one-third of this

TABLE 1[13]

Estimated Costs of Mental Illness (000's)

|  | 1963 | 1968 | 1971 | 1974 |
|---|---|---|---|---|
| Direct Costs | 2,401,700 | 4,030,974 | 11,058,299 | 1,693,059 |
| Indirect Costs | 4,634,000 | 16,906,000 | 14,179,382 | 19,812,768 |
| Total Costs | 7,035,700 | 20,936,974 | 25,237,681 | 21,805,827 |

amount to be associated with direct treatment costs[12] and two thirds with lack of productivity.

Direct costs include the care delivered in hospitals and out-patient facilities. Non-institutional care ranges from half-way and day-treatment facilities to vocational rehabilitation or private therapeutic services.

Indirect costs include a high death rate among schizophrenics, disability, reduced productivity, the suffering of families, and the cost of undesirable behavior attributable to mental illness. This cost was $19,812,786 in 1974.[14] This amount may be conservative due to a lack of readily available data and the operational difficulties in estimating indirect costs. For instance, while homicides or suicides may correlate with the incidence and prevalence of schizophrenia, specific and indicative data simply do not exist. Gunderson and Mosher in 1976 estimated the total loss of productivity from schizophrenia to be $10 billion per year[15] to the nation.

Statistical difficulties in determining the cost of chronic care include determining the number of people affected. But, given the lack of a generally accepted operational definition, alternatives have had to include definition by diagnosis or disability determination or by length of stay in a treatment facility or combinations thereof. Each approach risks miscalculation due to faulty and narrowly defined definitions.

A second difficulty in determining the cost of care is the lack of uniformity in reporting mechanisms which reflect variations in (definitions of) service, progress, cost accounting, or program configuration.

While the shift of patient care from institution to community has been well documented, actual transitions between the two have not. For example, some patients' needs are frequently not met in only one agency. Moreover, in the absence of a uniform reporting mechanism, changes in the number and nature of delivery sites complicate data reporting processes.

The cost of growing alternative living arrangements is also difficult to calculate. Cheap hotels, board-and-care homes, communal lodges, foster homes, and nursing homes each require different types of personnel; these costs, too, are not readily available. Moreover, long-term mentally disabled people not having experienced a recent hospitalization have not been included in data collection efforts.

In essence, multiple definitions, treatment modes, living arrangements, data systems, and loci of responsibility comprise the sources of problems in counting the schizophrenic population and estimating the direct and indirect costs of care.

Some efforts have been made to calculate the differences in cost between community and institutional care. In 1976, Sharfstein and Nafzeger found the cost of community care to be only 40% as expensive as the least expensive inpatient alternative.[16]

A second study[17] found the individual cost per patient to be the same whether a hospital or community-based program is used. More than 40% of the costs reflected other than direct treatment costs, such as inconveniences, family burden, or law enforcement.

Data gathered and analyzed by Gunderson and Mosher[18] suggest that the trend towards shorter hospitalization may actually increase the cost of schizophrenia to society. In comparing decrease in hospital treatment cost to the overall cost of providing a variety of services in the community, the latter cost is greater. They point out however, that hospital-centered treatment may limit the possibility of rehabilitation or the capacity to sustain paid employment.[19]

Gunderson and Mosher (1975) note that the available data may reflect a conservative bias due to the trends toward expensive private facilities, the rising cost of inpatient care, and the absence of data about the cost of private, outpatient visits.

Current trends in treatment cost reflect a variety of interrelated factors. The first of these is demographic. According to Gunderson and Mosher, 10-15 percent of all diagnosed schizophrenics will require long term care.[20] Most require several hospitalizations interspersed with prolonged periods of community living.

Two insurance-related factors have influenced patterns of community services for the non-hospitalized schizophrenic. The first is that insurance has played a less significant role in the funding of mental health programs than it has in funding general health services. The second is that insurance reimbursement for inpatient psychiatric units in general hospitals has not supported the development of partial hospitalization programs. For example, treatment in psychiatric hospitals has frequently been excluded by insurance coverage, or such care has provided only very limited benefits. However, funding for treatment of an inpatient psychiatric unit of a general hospital has been equivalent to the funding of care given in the medical or surgical units of the hospital, creating a bias favoring treatment in these units. These factors favor treatment in an inpatient psychiatric unit located in a general hospital.[21]

Juxtaposed with the concomitant trend towards community care, these policies leave the family victimized by contradictory policy impacts. On the one hand, the financial support of the schizophrenic is supplemented during periods of hospitalization. On the other hand, prompt release and community care are encouraged but are not supported either by the availability of appropriate facilities or by supplemental financial aid. One can deduce that while the patient is not hospitalized, the family is left with the obligation of providing appropriate living arrangements as well as financial and social supports to the schizophrenic member.

Between 1950 and 1970 the numbers of mentally ill in hospitals, as opposed to nursing home facilities, have reversed. That is, in 1950, 39% of institutionalized Americans were in mental health institutions and 19% were in nursing homes. Today the reverse is true: 44% are in nursing homes and 20% are in hospitals.[22] Recent studies indicate that 22% of the nursing home population is under age 65, and of these 20% are schizophrenic; nursing homes now represent at least 29% of mental health care for psychiatric inpatient care.

In addition to the shift from hospitals to community facilities and nursing home facilities, deinstitutionalization has resulted in still another trend. This trend has often been characterized as a "revolving door policy."[23] While there has been an unmistakable trend away from state hospitalizations, and while patients have been spending less time on the whole in the hospital, readmissions have nevertheless increased both in number and in proportion. In 1969, for instance, readmissions acounted for 49% of those entering state hospitals. By 1976, they constituted 57%.[24]

In some states, these figures rose from 43% in 1970 to 70% in 1974.[25] Hence, the revolving door.

One explanation for these trends is that funding options rather than the rhetoric of deinstitutionalization policies have driven the actual choice of living arrangements for schizophrenics. Families of schizophrenics may be choosing to hospitalize their ill members in order to help support them. Assuming that the schizophrenic is unable to care for him/herself, and that appropriate, non-institutional living arrangements are not available, the family is left with only two viable options. One choice is to care for the schizophrenic at home—often an untenable task due to the behavioral manifestations of the illness. The second is to locate available facilities that do offer financial support. Data cited earlier seem to indicate that families are opting for the latter choice—specifically for the use of nursing homes and revolving hospitalizations for the care and support of their schizophrenic member.

Twenty-three percent of the care of schizophrenia is covered by public insurance, including Medicare. State and local governments generally finance 31% of the total costs of mental illness. Private insurance plans cover 11% of the costs, while the individual or the family pay the remaining 35% of total costs. Based on the data in the Levine study, we have calculated that on the average this amounts to $1,500 per family per year.[26]

One can assume from these figures that upwards of one out of every three dollars spent on the care of schizophrenia is taken from the family. Out of the total cost estimate of $4.2 billion per year, $2.5 billion comes from the public sector,[27] while upwards of $1.5 billion comes from "out of pocket" family expenditures.

Given that more than one-third of the cost of the illness is financed by the family, one is in a position to make various assumptions. First is that the financial drain on families is severe. The family is caught between the Scylla of its sense of responsibility for its chronically dependent member; facing the family on the other side is the Charybdis of a burden it cannot afford. Second, patients from among less-than-upper-class families go without adequate care. Third, when services to patients are underfunded, services to vulnerable families are funded minimally, if at all.

Given the direct as well as the indirect costs of schizophrenia, one can draw other conclusions about the family as well. First, the family is left *de facto* to care for and support the vulnerable member, probably for the course of the patient's lifetime. Second, the family is not financially supported through public programs. Third, resources are not expected to support the vulnerable family at the same time it supports the vulnerable member. Currently, no public policy to share medical care costs or the costs of living arrangements or emotional support are available to help families of schizophrenics. While a patient lives in the community, the family is ultimately responsible for his or her care. Given the extreme stress that can be associated with caring for a severely disabled person, the lack of available support makes the family members of a schizophrenic an isolated, at-risk group.

## POLICY OPTIONS AND RECOMMENDATIONS

Policy options should include resources to support both patient and family. Because of the cyclical nature of the illness it makes sense for the family to function as orchestrator of available community services and, insofar as possible, as advocate for its vulnerable member. In this role, the family needs various supports; one is income support for hospitalization as needed as well as for home or community care. A second is emotional support so that the family does not become absorbed in the illness to the detriment of other family members. Support should be given to the development and socialization of each member of the vulnerable family, beginning with, but not limited to, the schizophrenic. The finances for such support should be one basis of an income policy for the vulnerable family.

Access and coordination of information systems must be coupled with clear diagnostic categories in order to determine the cost of care. What is evident is that long-term interventions are necessary and include direct treatment and psychological rehabilitation as well as income maintenance.

In summary, both the direct and indirect costs of schizophrenia to the patient and family should be supported by public policy. The role of the family should be specified and supported to include a leadership role in the care of the schizophrenic. However, no family should bear the sole burden of cost or care. The strength of the family and its members should be buttressed by a special income policy that would provide incentives for the family to help its schizophrenic member, but not hamper the development of other family members. Public resources should offer the family choice and access to community resources on an as-needed basis depending upon its assessment of the state of the patient and the needs of the members.

The major criticism of the deinstitutionalization movement has been that there are too few community services available to provide necessary services. Moreover, community services are tailored to meet acute needs rather than long-term needs.[28]

Nevertheless, federal and state initiatives are moving towards concentrated exploration of the use of community residences for the severely mentally disabled. At the same time, a trend towards the development and support of community support systems is evident. Residential alternatives offering multiple levels of treatment linked to a supportive network are preferred objectives.

Legitimization is the second major challenge. The community residence, born outside the mental health system, must interface with the community and satisfy appropriate concerns such as quality control, building codes, and zoning requirements. A carefully and judiciously developed standard will be a distinct asset to the entire range of interested parties—client, provider, state legislature, and national bodies; standards will help to counter abuse, unsafe facilities, discrimination, and fiscal mismanagement.[29]

Studies of psychiatric disorders have found that only a fraction of all people with debilitating symptoms actually receive treatment from mental health professionals. Most, according to several studies, tend to turn first to clergymen, lawyers, or the police.[30]

Alternatives to hospitalizing the long-term or chronic patient can be developed within a system of community mental health programs when that system makes a commitment to a total population and develops a variety of direct and indirect services for chronic as well as acute patients. But the special needs of the chronically ill need to be identified and kept within an overall system rather than within a single project. When the system includes an evaluative component it is possible to define needs, develop programs, and assess the outcome of programs in a manner which permits modification and further planning.

Obviously, the primary focus must be the patient. Optimal treatment options must include a variety of living patterns. These should follow the patient from pre-hospital services to aftercare or rehabilitation. Likewise, living settings should vary from pre-hospital to independent living. Second, coordinated mechanisms must be devised regarding funding patterns. Treatment and housing options should be flexible and should reflect patient needs rather than funding-source-accountability requirements.

Assisting the schizophrenic to be independent is the best possible support available to the family. Otherwise, it is the family who is continually saddled with the long-term role of unsupported provider. That is, if there are no community facilities available, the patient may be more likely to turn to his/her nuclear family for support. Support obviously includes the provision of a home.

Because of the disorderly behavior of many schizophrenics, it may not be in the best interest of the patient or other family members for the patient to live at home. The patient needs professional care which the family cannot provide. Also, a family home cannot service as a treatment center. Patients often lose track of time; often they forget to attend to such details as snuffing burning cigarettes. Thus, in addition to causing emotional strain, a patient can be disruptive during sleeping hours and pose real threats to physical property.

Frequently, an element of collusion may be found when a patient who demonstrates a need for professional help stays at home. He/she is less likely to seek professional help or seek new levels of independence if family surroundings are available. At the same time, the normal household routine and personal relationships can be severely taxed while a severely disturbed person is in the home. Thus, the vulnerable family without benefit of professional support becomes more vulnerable by virtue of the stress imposed upon it by the constant presence of a schizophrenic member.

We lack a national policy which states that families must take care of all of their members *or* that families will be relieved of explicit responsibilities under the particular circumstances which severe mental illness can present. On the other hand, it is generally held that the family does constitute a fundamental social institution which needs to be sustained, that it constitutes the most flexible social service of first resort. At the same time, there is widespread acceptance of the belief that the family is overburdened in specific areas, that it needs to be relieved, and that this relief should be primarily provided by public intervention.

The many and sometimes contradictory views through which society perceives mental illness and the role of families in which it occurs is dramatically evident in the case of schizophrenia. Both the lack of resources made available to the schizophrenic and his

Figure 1

HOSPITALIZATION OPTIONS FROM MOST TO LEAST RESTRICTIVE

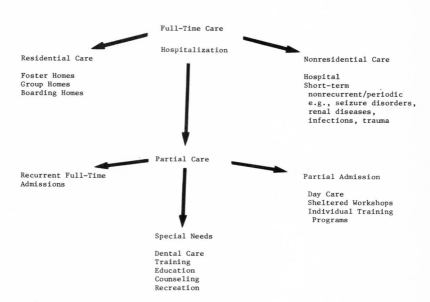

Full-Time Care

Hospitalization

Residential Care

Foster Homes
Group Homes
Boarding Homes

Nonresidential Care

Hospital
Short-term
    nonrecurrent/periodic
    e.g., seizure disorders,
    renal diseases,
    infections, trauma

Partial Care

Recurrent Full-Time
Admissions

Partial Admission

Day Care
Sheltered Workshops
Individual Training
    Programs

Special Needs

Dental Care
Training
Education
Counseling
Recreation

or her family, and the confusion surrounding the concept of patients' rights have indicated ambiguity, mediocre care, and an absence of preventive intervention for families. In this regard, this paper has provided an overview of schizophrenia as it produces, and then negatively impacts, a vulnerable family and vulnerable member.

With the advent of the Social Security Act, and, more recently, the Supplemental Security Income program, the mentally disabled, along with other groups, have had access to some independent sources of health care and income. This access symbolically reinforces the already apparent tendency of families to live in separate nuclear units, since these benefits are less available to schizophrenics living at home.

As a society, we seem to be moving increasingly in the direction of shifting fiscal responsibility from the family to state. Under

SSI, for example, policies regarding filial responsibility are within the purview of the state. By 1979 many states made no demands on families, but 21 others did not make assistance grants contingent upon such contribution. Since the remainder of states take into account the income level of potential contributing family members, the degree of family responsibility is even further reduced.

Since most families have incomes of less than $17,000 annually, there are relatively few cases in which there is a sufficient disposable margin of family income to make feasible a demand that payments be made for the support of patients living elsewhere. On one hand, it can be said that the precept that families take care of their dependent family member has been somewhat invaded, and that as a practical matter, families are relieved of this responsibility. On the other hand, given a paucity of policy supports and extant resources, the family continues to be *de facto* responsible for its schizophrenic member.

Recognition of this dilemma has been obscured because of the distinctions made between public assistance and social security. The stigma of public assistance and the existence of a two-tier assistance system has encouraged the maintenance of the traditional societal view of family relationships. But on the other hand, the introduction of disability under SSI relieves the family somewhat of its ongoing responsibility for its schizophrenic member.

In the past, furthermore, we have stressed concern for the vulnerable and rejected child. But looking at family policy from the point of view of the schizophrenic, a disturbing situation has occurred. On one hand, the family is perceived as the bulwark and sovereign power with respect to family needs. On the other hand, families are incapable of dealing with continual chronic disability. The financial and psychosocial burdens are too intense.

The reasons for the inadequacy of community-based services for schizophrenics seem to be manifold. In addition to insufficient funds, some of the frequently cited factors include: 1) treatment objectives based upon cure rather than stabilization; 2) lack of motivation of staff to work with chronic patients because the intrinsic rewards are few and the work particularly demanding; 3) inadequate training of mental health professionals, including poor modelling by faculty in training institutions; 4) insufficient attention to continuity of care; and 5) inappropriate use of treatment models designed for healthier outpatients.[31]

In addition to inadequate community facilities, protective and developmental care of the mentally disabled is lacking an effective model for intervention. Specifically, the traditional mode of therapy has as its objective improvement which may be, by definition of the illness, impossible. What is needed is a treatment model that acknowledges prognosis but addresses community adjustment through the development of skills needed to 1) acquire material resources such as food, shelter, clothing, and social service benefits; 2) to acquire coping skills such as using public transportation or preparing and budgeting for everyday living matters such as preparing nutritious meals; 3) to acquire motivation to strive for a network of people with whom to interact.

What schizophrenic patients in the community need is support and the development of basic living skills to keep them free from hospitalization for as long as possible but with access to hospitalization on a revolving door, as-needed basis. On this level, the care of the patient is, in effect, support for the family. If the patient is cared for in the community, other family members are free to pursue their own growth and development.

Another way of characterizing the crucial problem of cost for caring for the mentally ill is that we have not devised a mechanism whereby funding follows patients regardless of the type of care they are receiving. For example, as patients have been relocated from hospital to day treatment or community settings, no concomitant shift in funding has occurred. Similarly, while the schizophrenic person might receive Medicaid reimbursement for treatment costs while in a nursing home, they are not eligible for reimbursement while in a hospital. Patients living in apartment programs and single-room occupancy hotels are eligible for SSI but these benefits are not applicable to institutional settings. In essence, patients are shifted from hospital to nursing home or to welfare hotel, and monies are not available for follow-up care. Thus, the family is left with the cost of providing access and referral to needed service.

The requirements for each funding agency are different with regard to benefits, benefit levels, and eligibility requirements. Money is provided for programs rather than for people requiring flexible movement from one program or system of programs into another. Despite the allocation of millions of federal dollars for the mentally ill, dollars flow in a haphazard manner by program— i.e., housing, medical care, income maintenance—rather than by the needs of particular individuals.

One way of capturing the disjointed aspect of community care for the schizophrenic is to note that there is an inadequate range of facilities for the mentally ill in the community. Each type of program is designed for a specific level of need, that is for the individuals with different problems or levels of functioning. But, because of a lack of access and referral mechanisms and because of an overall lack of facilities, patients are placed in facilities on the basis of geographical convenience regardless of whether they are appropriate sites of care. No level of government assumes responsibility for coordination of care for the patient after his release from the hospital.

Nor are adequate rehabilitation and preparation programs provided for patients as they are about to be released from hospitals. With neither adequate preparation for re-entry into the community nor adequate community support, it is no wonder that readmission rates are high and success rates are low. Coupled with community resistance to establishing community facilities, patients are left very much on their own resources.

The trend towards de-institutionalization has outlined in bold relief that the patients remaining in hospitals are chronic mental patients. They are not ordinary citizens suffering from acute schizophrenic breaks that subside. These are people suffering from impaired social functioning. We lack a model of care for people for whom the concept of cure is for practical purposes meaningless. We also lack a model of support for their families. We offer cure but not care to people who desperately need the latter and for which the former does not exist at this time.

In essence, if future studies continue to demonstrate the economic and human benefits of community care, those responsible for allocating private and public resources will have to respond by funding community programs more adequately. Moreover, to be effective, staff will have to be trained, supported, and rewarded for the intense and often intrinsically non-rewarding nature of day-by-day work with chronic schizophrenics.

Integration of schizophrenics with community life can only take place within an atmosphere of neighborhood and family acceptance coupled with extensive policy support and professional intervention. As Budson points out (p. 210), residential programs are currently caught between funding inadequacies, a piece-meal community delivery system that is in transition, a lack of legislative appropriations, and community opposition to integration.

In the final analysis, the strongest support for the family of a schizophrenic is a coordinated system of community care for the ill person. The burden of the vulnerable family can be alleviated, given the appropriate financial, living, and supportive arrangements discussed in the body of this paper. Also, the public provision of decent assistance symbolizes support for the family to share its burden with the state and not be continuously overwhelmed or hemmed in by it.

## NOTES AND REFERENCES

1. *President's Commission on Mental Health*, Thomas E. Bryant, Chairperson. Washington, D.C. Superintendent of Documents, 1978, Vol. II, p. 18.

2. Martha Ozawa and Duncan Lindsley, "Schizophrenia and SSI II," *Social Work*, March, 1979.

3. *President's Commission on Mental Health*, op. cit., Vol. II, p. 18.

4. Herbert Weiner, "Schizophrenia: Etiology," in Alfred M. Freedman, Harold I. Kaplan and Benjamin J. Sadock, ed., *Comprehensive Textbook of Psychiatry*, 2nd ed., Baltimore: Williams and Wilkins, 1975, p. 876.

5. Loren E. Mosher, "Schizophrenics, Recent Trends," in Freedman et al., op. cit., pp. 982-991.

6. D. Rosenthal and S.S. Kety, "An Essay on Psychoanalytic Theory: Two Theories of Schizophrenia," *International Journal of Psychoanalysis*, 4, 1973.

7. Heinz Lehman, "Psychotic Disorders," in Freedman, Kaplan and Sadock, op. cit., pp. 851-859.

8. Sigmund Freud, "The Case of Schriber," in *Standard Edition of the Complete Works of Sigmund Freud*, London: Hogarth Press, 1958, Vol. 12, p. 3 as quoted in Lehman op. cit., p. 856.

9. M. Klein, *Contributions of Psychoanalysis, 1921-1945*, London: Hogarth, 1950, and H.S. Sullivan, *The Interpersonal Theory of Psychiatry*, New York: W.W. Norton, 1953.

10. Theodore Lidz, "The Family, Language and the Transmission of Schizophrenia" and L. Wynne, "Methodologic and Conceptual Issues in the Study of Schizophrenics and Their Families," in D. Rosenthal and S.S. Kety, eds., *The Transmission of Schizophrenia*, Oxford: Pergamon Press, 1968.

11. John A. Talbott, *Death of the Asylum*, New York, Guire and Stratton, 1979, p. 37.

12. John G. Gunderson and Loren Mosher, "Cost of Schizophrenia," *American Journal of Psychiatry*, September 1975, pp. 901-906.

13. Steven Sharfstein and Harry W. Clark, "Economics and the Chronic Mental Patient," *Schizophrenia Bulletin* 4 (1978), p. 399.

14. Ibid.

15. Gunderson and Mosher arrive at this figure by taking a prevalence rate of 2-3% for schizophrenia, by assuming that 75% of schizophrenics are unemployed, and calculating a yearly income of $5,000 by taking one-fourth of the national average for a four-person family ($10,000 corrected downward). See Gunderson and Mosher, op. cit., p. 902.

16. Steven Sharfstein and J. Nafzeger, "Community Care: Costs and Benefits for a Chronic Patient," *Hospital and Community Psychiatry*, 27 (3), 1976, pp. 170-173.

17. Burton A. Weisbrod, "A Guide to Benefit-Cost Analysis As Seen Through A Controlled Experiment in Treating the Mentally Ill," Madison, Wisconsin: University of Wisconsin, Institute for Research on Poverty Discussion Paper #559-79.

18. Gunderson and Mosher, op. cit., p. 902.

19. Ibid., p. 905.

20. Ibid. p. 903.

21. Raymond F. Luber, ed., *Partial Hospitalization*, New York: Plenum Press, 1979.

22. Talbott, op. cit. p. 36.

23. John A. Talbott, "Stopping the Revolving Door Policy: A Study of Readmissions to a State Hospital," *Psychiatric Quarterly* 48 (1974), pp. 159-168.

24. Talbott, *Death of the Asylum*, op. cit., p. 39.

25. Government Accounting Office, *Returning the Mentally Disabled to the Community: Government Needs to Do More*, Washington, D.C.: January 1977.

26. Dan and Dianne Levine, "The Cost of Mental Illness," DHEW Publication Adm #76-265, Washington, D.C.: Superintendent of Documents, 1971.

27. *President's Commission on Mental Health*, op. cit.

28. S. Colton and I. Sterling, "Community Residential Treatment Strategies," *Community Mental Health Review* 3 (September-December 1978), p. 1.

29. Richard D. Budson, *The Psychiatric Halfway House: A Handbook of Theory and Practice*, Pittsburgh: University of Pittsburgh Press, 1978.

30. B. Dohrenwend, "The Attitude of Local Leaders Toward Behavioral Disorder," in Bruce Dohrenwend and Lawrence Kolb, eds, *Urban Challenges to Psychiatry*, Boston: Little Brown, 1969.

31. L. I. Test and M.A. Stein, "An Alternative to Mental Hospital Treatment," in L.I. Stein and M.A. Test, *Alternatives to Mental Hospital Treatment*, New York: Plenum Press, 1978.

# PART IV: POLICY DIRECTIONS

# Introduction to Part IV

This final section begins with a paper by Robert Morris, who poses the critical policy choices concerning family home care. He positions his discussion in relation to the current questioning of the accomplishments and the costs of the Welfare State. Assuming the necessity for a public program of aid to care-giving families, Morris asks how this can be done without emptying the public purse, a consideration that has concerned politicians and public alike since the Elizabethan statutes tried to protect the treasury by requiring families to be responsible for "every poor, old, blind, lame and impotent person." The paper goes on to consider who should be given priority in the allocation of public resources for long term care: the poor, people without families, or all families who meet certain criteria of need.

Morris examines the most promising avenues of innovation—cash grants, social insurance, new types of agencies and service programs—but also asks whether we should be cautious and first make incremental improvements in existing programs. As he moves further into the means of providing home care, Morris deals with two important questions—who should control the flow of resources: consumers, professionals, or public functionaries—and where will the personnel come from to perform the paraprofessional tasks necessary to assist families in caring for their disabled relatives.

Against the background of the demographic realities that make home care both so necessary and so problematic, Morris proposes principles and criteria by which to choose our policies.

In the chapter taken from *Family Care of the Elderly*, Frank-father and his colleagues draw upon the lessons of the Family

Support Program (FSP) they studied in New York, giving careful attention to the practicalities of implementation in outlining a "home-care entitlement" program for the chronically disabled. While the FSP served elderly, disabled people with and without family resources and those living with or apart from their families, the researchers recommend a program that addresses many of the critical operational and definitional problems with which this book is concerned, e.g., how much can society expect of families and how much and what kinds of supportive services should be extended to them without weakening the tremendous contribution they now make to care of the disabled.

The FSP researchers propose a maintenance model which provides for user control of benefits and standardized determinations of eligibility and of benefit levels based on disability tests, in preference to the more prevalent professional model which stresses diagnosis, treatment, and rehabilitation.

Following these papers is a brief note by the editor describing the use of the tax system to assist care-giving families financially. The volume closes with some concluding observations by the editor.

# Caring for Vulnerable Family Members: Alternative Policy Options

Robert Morris

Any discussion of alternative policies concerning the family is bound to be an untidy effort. Sharply defined alternatives are likely to appear oversimplified, and those which seek to comprehend the complexity of this subject are likely to end up being vague and inconclusive. If we define a social policy as a guiding principle, or set of principles, with which government deals with present and future uncertainties, then there appear to be four major types of policies we can consider to meet non-medical services for the severely handicapped (personal care, bathing, feeding, mobility, etc.) as well as providing medical and hospital care.

1. Families, however defined, can be expected to care for all of their members by their own labor or by purchase: this view has persisted over the millenia and is still widely held although, as a guiding principle, it has been invaded and eroded from the earliest historical times. Mutual aid and various acts of government have from the earliest times helped families and their troubled members—at least in extreme conditions of distress.

2. Public or collective responsibility might be assumed for all vulnerable family members. In this extreme form, this has hardly ever been proposed seriously although, for sharply limited types of vulnerability, almost universal public responsibility has become a reality, at least in advanced industrial states: the very severely mentally retarded and the very neurologically disabled have long been cared for in publicly supported institutions with minimum demands made upon family members. Since the 1930s there has also been an increasing tendency for public programs to take over responsibility for aged members of families, at least if they have— at the time of their need—been living outside of homes of other relatives. Few states have very strong or enforceable filial support legislation.

3. Case-negotiated programming represents a third set of op-

tions. Here, the innumerable varieties of family circumstances and personal conditions are viewed as inappropriate for any standardized approach. Instead reliance is placed upon expert professional judgment, be it that of the physician, the psychiatrist, the social worker, or nurse, who will decide when a public program becomes applicable and for what individuals and families, and the degree of family responsibility which can be relied upon. In recent years, this approach has attracted a wide professional support behind concepts of case management and case assessment for admission into public programs.

4. Finally, a policy of shared responsibility between the state and family can be contemplated. In this option, it is not a question of all responsibility to the family or all to the state. Instead, programs and policies are designed which permit the state to supplement and complement family responsibility, but in a clear and unambiguous fashion not dependent upon individual case negotiation. Demogrants and aid-in-attendance allowances are illustrative of this approach, although it has not been widely adopted in the U.S. In it, at a minimum, some financial assistance is provided whenever an individual is identified as having a specified vulnerable condition, but this amount is seldom sufficient to meet all the needs of that individual. Rather, it is assumed that family members, friends, and others will complement or supplement this basic minimum so that the two act together in a symbiotic relationship.

## DIFFICULTIES IN MAKING CHOICES

Examining these options and making choices among them in any operational sense is most difficult for a number of reasons. First, there is the underlying lack of agreement about what constitutes a family. Acknowledging that new forms of family structure are being experimented with in many parts of the world, structures not legalized by religion or law and including relationships among individuals of the same sex—with or without children—still some meaningful definition is necessary if we are to talk about policy as action of government. For my purposes, I believe the "family" is that collectivity of individuals bound together by some reasonably explicit ties which involve mutual rights and obligations among the members of the collectivity, and which rights and obligations are expected to persist over time. In this formulation, and I recognize that it is not universally accepted, the focus of family policy, *qua* family policy, is on the collectivity, not upon the individual members thereof. True, what happens to individual members in the collectivity becomes a variable which affects the choice of policy, but the policy in the end needs to be viewed not from the point of view of individual members but of the collectivity.

Policy is also obscured because we simply do not know whether the dynamics of family relationships, however defined, are governed by a basic, fundamental desire of family members to care for each other when they can, or whether the basic dynamic is to divest the collectivity of responsibility for members who become vulnerable. We no longer tolerate the practice of some primitive societies to isolate disabled members and allow them to die without food or support of any kind. But neither are we completely comfortable with the idea that families normally take care of all their members regardless of the burden which it places upon the other members. It is not so much a matter of what we think "should exist," but what is the underlying dynamic which drives family members to care for each other. Depending upon our understanding, we can devise policies which reinforce the basic direction of these underlying dynamics, or we can seek to impose a contrary, normative standard in the interests of the society.

Next, we need to recognize that public policy for the family is only one of numerous examples of the dilemma confronting the liberal tradition in the western world. There has in recent years emerged a very great doubt about the capacity of society to care well for its members in an organized public sense over time. Numerous publications have of late probed this period of uncertainty.[1] An oversimplified summation of this criticism of the liberal welfare state ideal runs somewhat as follows: In the U.S., certainly since the middle-1930s, there has been an expanding belief that government—meaning the state—has an obligation to provide care and to provide resolution of an ever-widening range of human difficulties going far beyond the conventional prevention of starvation and including today the absolute guarantee of a minimum level of income, the management of a wide variety of mental illnesses and peculiarities in behavior, and the shaping of the family.

In order to carry out these widening obligations, it has for some decades been assumed that publicly administered or financed programs, delivered through formal agencies or handled by cash payments to individuals, are all affected by a generally benevolent and caring attitude on the part of the providers. However, this approach has also required that the providers be given increasing levels of power and authority in order to carry out their assigned tasks. As the tasks have become more complex and more variegated, so have increased the levels of authority which are assigned to the state and to providers to make judgments, to intervene, and to act in the lives of many individuals. With time, it has appeared that this increase in power and authority has been abused as often as not, and it is widely questioned whether public programs can be helpful to individuals without at the same time controlling their lives, and becoming in effect tyrants over the lives of innumerable members of society. The behaviors of public assistance staffs, of mental hospital and nursing home personnel, of psychiatrists administering drugs, and of housing authorities—to name but a few—have all been subjected to this criticism.

The fact that professionals and professionalization have also increased their role and authority in this system has done little to mitigate the criticisms. Instead, professionalization itself has been frequently accused of being unfeeling and given to professional aggrandizement rather than sensitivity to the needs of recipients. The net effect of these attacks coming not only from the die-hard conservatives, but from the most liberal and radical members in the public policy arena, has placed the liberal center in substantial jeopardy, lacking a sense of confidence or direction.

Illustrative of this malaise are such quotations as these:

> Consumerism . . . increases the material consumption (and) only creates demands for more indulgence.

> The difficulties of the welfare state cannot be resolved by increases in supply alone; a restructuring of the demand for social welfare is required.

> Enabling legislation and agency practice enhanced the prerogatives of state officials and reduced—almost eliminated—legal protection and rights of those coming under their authority.

> We are witnessing the dissolution of the Progressive version of community as a viable concept, indeed the breakdown of normality as a viable concept . . . not only can no one agree on what is good for all of us . . . The perspective

is not the perspective of common welfare but the needs of the
particular group. The intellectual premises are not unity but
conflict. It is "us" versus "them." (organize one's own special
interest group).

Can we do good to others but on their terms?[2]


Even where these deep-seated doubts are not accepted, there
still remains a substantial uncertainty about the capacity of public
organization to discriminate in any fine-tuned fashion as it admin-
isters generally benign and benevolent programs without at the
same time introducing a large measure of discrimination. This
critique comes in large part as a result of the operation of our
open and widening political system. We have come to expect that
minorities of many kinds will be the beneficiaries of programs,
but the resources have always been limited. As a result, programs
intended for the most vulnerable classes have been required just
as much by members of the middle class. The feeble and disabled
grandparent or parent, the alcoholic, the abused child, the mentally
ill person, are found just as frequently among the middle class
as among the poor and minorities. Programs have inevitably had to
spread themselves to accommodate a class of conditions regardless
of economic or social status. The idea that the poorest have less
capacity (in an economic or in a moral sense) to look after their
members than do the middle class has obviously been substantially
altered, and by now the question of family responsibility is no
longer a matter of class or economic status, even though middle-
class families do have more economic means and more security
with which to cope with many difficulties. The consequence has
been a thinning out of resources to meet much wider demand.
But it is not just a matter of income or class. Programs have
not been able to fine-tune very well the normal professional desire
to concentrate on curative efforts rather than caring for the vulnerable. As a result, almost all public and private programs concentrate
whatever resources they have on the more hopeful cases and generally tend to neglect the most severe cases where the opportunity
for cure is reduced.
These doubts about what constitutes the family, about the basic
family dynamics concerning the vulnerable, and doubts about society's capacity to either care well for anyone over time or, if it
does provide this care, to do so in any fine-tuned fashion, consti-

tute only a few of the grave difficulties we confront as we try to make policy choices.

## SOME DEMOGRAPHIC REALITIES

Fortunately, there are a few demographic realities which provide a reasonably firm foundation with which to examine policy alternatives. Briefly, these are the following:

1. The first and perhaps the most significant and yet little-recognized phenomenon is this: nationally, about 20% of all older persons have no living children. A recent Harris Poll finds that over 22% of urban elderly have no living children, 16% of suburban elderly, nearly 22% of small-town elderly, and over 17% of rural elderly have no living children.[3] Bane reports that persons over 65 in 1970 were members of a generation born around the turn of the century, a period of low marriage rates and high rates of childlessness. It is likely that this circumstance has not substantially altered today where we find that the reduced number of children born to families, the relatively high proportion of persons never married, and the frequency of divorce which, even when it is succeeded by a subsequent marriage, may attenuate the bonds of long-term family responsibility, add up to a situation in which the kith and kin network continues to be diminished in its extensiveness and in its commitment to all members. There are fewer adult children, aunts, cousins, and the like. I have stressed the position of the elderly without family, or without children at least, because they constitute perhaps half of the social problem complex with which our subject must concern itself. The situation is less dramatic when it comes to children, for the amount of orphanage has been substantially reduced in the past hundred years.

2. The second demographic reality is closely linked to that most surprising, unplanned economic and cultural phenomenon—the virtual disappearance of family manpower for the performance of family tasks. For some decades, the wishes and aspirations of most individuals in our society have combined with the requirements of an industrial economy to lead almost all adult family members to seek paid employment outside of the family. The proportion of married men and women who are simultaneously employed has been enlarged by the flood into the labor market of teenagers who consider themselves deprived if there is not a job during the summer holiday, immediately upon graduation from

school, or even part-time work during their school years. This phenomenon is noted without a value being placed upon it. In a society where the wishes of the individual are paramount, this may provide a maximum opportunity for self-realization. However, in a society concerned with a collectivity known as the family, it is important to recognize that family manpower to carry out many remaining tasks within the family has almost disappeared as a result of this trend.

If there is available manpower, it consists of male youth (mainly minority), not the unattached female who performed what has been historically identified as "woman's work." Can incentives convert age long prejudices about suitable roles for boys and girls?

It is important to note that our information on this subject may be somewhat distorted by a preoccupation with the dominant middle class representing perhaps 80% of the population. That approximately 20% which is not only poor at intervals, but poor throughout life and likely to be on some kind of assistance, may have a different set of values.

Recent studies of AFDC recipients suggest that this population, by and large, has concerns outside of the main achieving stream of the rest of society, that working outside the home is not as highly valued as looking after the household and the family within the home, and that these individuals have developed their own set or network of institutions such as the evangelical storefront churches which give moral structure and meaning to their lives.

3. Finally, there are the fragments of information about who does care, at least for the elderly now, which may give us some base points for future action. For example, where there are adult children for the elderly, on average about 55% of the elderly have had a face-to-face contact with their adult children within the past day or two, and an additional 25.5% have had an additional contact within the last week.[4] The same sources indicate that about 70% of the elderly receive help from adult children when they are ill, 34% have the children running errands for them or fixing things around the house, and 91% receive gifts. When it comes to physical assistance, perhaps the most meaningful measure of family care for the vulnerable, it is important to note that in the Harris Poll over 40% on average of the elderly receive no help from adult children. There is some variation here, for the older persons—especially the widowed—are more likely to receive this

physical assistance either from adult children or their neighbors if they live in rural rather than urban communities.

These various sources suggest that families which have a higher income and higher education tend to provide more care or financial support and to do more for their vulnerable members, when they are located in nursing homes or similar institutions. These families are somewhat less likely to provide this kind of care in their own homes.

## THE EVOLUTION OF PUBLIC POLICY FOR VULNERABLE PERSONS

A reasonable reading of the evolution of welfare policy suggests that from the very earliest times of recorded history there has been some form of public responsibility assumed for the most vulnerable in society: the very badly crippled, the widow, and the orphan. The 20th century has seen a very great and continuing enlargement of the concept of vulnerability, resulting in what is commonly identified as the welfare state. In the U.S., for example, it is not only widows or orphaned children or the permanently disabled who are considered "worthy" or entitled to public attention. All able-bodied persons without work are entitled to some assistance. Sick and crippled children, those with developmental disabilities, the retarded, and those with neurological handicaps are entitled to public help at least for curative and rehabilitation purposes, frequently without regard to family capacity or status. The aged, regardless of family position, are now assured of minimum income and medical care through Social Security insurance, and, where this is not sufficient, become entitled to additional assistance with only minimal filial responsibility. True, the public assistance aspect of this enlargement of responsibility is frequently cruel and harsh, requiring that the older person who is living away from adult children virtually pauperize himself and spend down to an eligible level, consuming all of his assets and removing the sense of security which derives from having some assets available. But this enlargement of the concept of vulnerability does not stop here. The state is actively involved in "doing something" about children whose education is unsatisfactory or who are poorly achieving in school; it tries feebly to do something about the worst kinds of housing. The mentally ill, or perhaps the person described as "acting peculiarly," is entitled to "treatment" to get him to conform to whatever the social norm may be in his community, or is institutionalized in order to prevent his peculiarities being too evident to other more "normally behaving" members of society.

It is clear that the concept of vulnerability as regards public responsibility has been exponentially enlarged in the 20th century. Gronbjerg[5] has argued that with the 20th century, and in industrialized westernized states, has come an increasing participation in political affairs by more and more citizens and more and more special interest groups. As a result, civil and political citizenship which was ideologically a product of the 18th and 19th centuries has been followed very closely in the 20th century by what Marshall has called social citizenship, that is, "the whole range from the right to a modicum of economic welfare and security to the right to share to the full in the social heritage of a civilized being according to the standards prevailing in this society.[6] This enlarged participation Gronbjerg calls the mass society accompanied by mass education, mass communication, and a wide diffusion of culture at the center. As a result, a kind of civil equality between the elite and the masses has resulted, producing the welfare state. This in turn underpins the current belief in individual rights to self-realization in lieu of family obligation.

In this circumstance, the old idea of the "deserving" poor, used in a moral sense, has now been enormously widened to contain many who are considered "helpless enough," which is a social evaluation subject to constant change.

This evolution, however, has taken place while a very deep uncertainty in mass perception and consciousness persists. Much of the ethical mooring of the "normal" citizen may still be in the 18th century when it was assumed that we care publicly for a few of the obviously vulnerable persons, such as the crippled and the orphaned, but not for others who are really the responsibility of the family and the individual. Thus, the ideas about the scope of public responsibility conflict with the ideas about individual freedom to realize the self so characteristic of the mass society of the 20th century. No clear, ethical foundation thus exists for deciding what is the obligation of the individual, let alone an obligation of the family collective for its own members. The obverse of this statement, of course, is that there is public uncertainty about the extent of public responsibility.

One result of this set of contradictions has been well-described by Murray Edelman, who has argued that generally such contradictions result in words that succeed and policies that fail.[7] Chronic problems which force policymakers and their constituencies to confront contradictory beliefs and chronic problems lead them to utilize a language which promises much and policies which are bound to fail since they do not succeed in reconciling either the chronicity or the contradictions which underlie the policy dilemmas. We straddle the dilemmas by a resort to high rhetoric and failed policies.

## SOME POLICY ALTERNATIVES—WHO IS TO BE HELPED

In discussing some policy alternatives, I hope to consider a few which are reasonably feasible, rather than concentrating on certain alternatives which, while rhetorically satisfying, are unlikely to be realized in the present political situation. Those I think unreal are ones which argue that the state has full responsibility for all vulnerable persons and thus relieves the family completely when any burden arises; or, conversely, that all of these burdens rest entirely with the family.

For purely personal reasons, perhaps of prejudice, I will not spend much time on the case-negotiated option. In this option we rely mainly on physicians, sometimes on social workers, to discuss wants with clients. The professional then prescribes what is to be recommended based on a mix of expert judgment about what is needed, expert knowledge of what is available, and what the client will accept. The recommendation is limited by what a family is able and willing to spend its own resources on; or lacking income, it is limited by what is already being provided for by a social program. Mal-allocation of public resources and prejudices in expert judgment seriously flaw this method, widespread though it is. It is widely available and widely understood. However, I believe cumulative evidence suggests that professional judgments are as frequently flawed as not and that it would be undesirable to build a policy which relies primarily upon final judgments being made by professionals over the daily lives of too many other persons.

This leads me to concentrate on that fourth set of options where some division of shared responsibility between the family and the state, the family as a collective and the state (meaning government) can be shaped.

1. *Helping the poor*. Here, I mean the economically poor. This is the system we essentially have now with all of its deficiencies. It is carried by Medicaid and SSI or their variants. It retains a two-tier system of provision; the assumption here is that the middle-class family (and I avoid the thorny difficulty of where to draw the line of middle class) is assumed capable of caring for its vulnerable family members *where there is a family*. They can provide this care themselves through their own efforts, or can pay for the purchase of service whether provided by public or private providers. In this option, it is the poor who are unable to manage for simple economic reasons. If the family income is too low and all members are working, as our society seems to encourage, then the combined earned income is still not sufficient to purchase supportive help and, therefore, public intervention is necessary either in the form of a directly provided service or money to the poor to purchase on a basis more or less comparable to that of the middle class. If, on the other hand, a family is poor and all the members are not working, such a policy would assume that the family members provide the care themselves. This may be highly inequitable, for in these same circumstances middle-class families have the option of either providing the care or buying it from others, which is not made available to the poor who are not employed. Such a policy seems to be inequitable, but probably widely acceptable to the conservative elements of the electorate.

2. *Concentrate on members of society who have no family*. Obviously, implementing such a policy requires clarifying who constitutes a family member; but, in the conventional sense, this would mean at the minimum persons without either parents or adult children. Although identifying who lacks a family probably has a great deal of ambiguity about it, it is doubtful whether the ambiguities are as great as those which surround present definitions of entitlement to public assistance or support. Such a policy would bear heavily upon intact families, however they are defined, and would probably bear even more heavily upon individuals who do have a family but where the family is uncaring or completely rejecting. Its only virtue is that the target population is relatively easy to identify and it is also clear that this population without family members is, without question, the most necessitous of all vulnerable persons. An individual who has any condition con-

sidered vulnerable—be it illness, disability, or whatever—and who
has no relative to whom he can turn for counsel, encouragement,
or help is clearly the most deprived of all human beings. Responsibility of the state for these members of society would seem
to be unchallengeable and unquestioned. Perhaps this represents
a minimum rock-bottom of public responsibility upon which can
be built other kinds of responsibility for those with overburdened
families or whose families are rejecting.

3. *A third approach* would base public programs on help to
any family, regardless of economic condition, where a specified
condition or group of conditions is found to exist. Just what conditions are to be included—be they a given level of disability,
a given level of deviant behavior, or whatnot—a substantial bu-
reaucratic and professional apparatus is necessary to make the
assessment and judgment. There is substantial precedent for this.
The Social Security system uses such a mechanism to identify
an insured member who is so severely and permanently disabled
as to warrant early entitlement to income replacement (that is,
retirement income replacement, not disability income); all medical
programs rely on physician judgments about who enters the hospital; all medical programs rely upon clerical intermediaries to
decide whether reimbursement for particular conditions fall within
the guidelines; and the Veterans Administration has a long experience in deciding what level of disability warrants what level of
financial assistance or attendant allowance. The major question
here is whether as a society we trust the state sufficiently to turn
over so large a measure of authority to professional bureaucracies.
If we decide that we can, then the major dilemmas are identifying
the conditions to be covered and the nature of the sliding scale
whereby more economically secure families at least contribute
some part of the cost.

Some cautions need to be introduced, however, before we adopt
too readily what seems to be a reasonable policy. Most of the
tasks with which we will have to deal are unpleasant ones. The
vulnerable conditions are not the ones which respond to medical
or rehabilitative therapy in a reasonable period of time; they are
the problems which persist over time and for which individuals
require a great deal of physical care and patience. It is just these
unpleasant tasks which families as well as social agencies and
medical institutions prefer to off-load to someone else, given an
opportunity. We need to recognize that about 80% of all caring

tasks are now extended by family members to their vulnerable parties when there is a family at all. This approach would therefore involve a very great increase in public expenditure. Enlarged Medicare or health insurance could be the vehicles.

Numerous estimates suggest that about 12% of the elderly require some kind of supplementary help if they are living outside of institutions. Between one-third and one-half now get some kind of public help of a limited nature. One can estimate that the increase, over time, in demand would widen this gap between the present proportion now getting assistance and the estimated total believed to need such supplementary help, unless remedial steps are taken.

Finally, it is important to ask ourselves what is the source of manpower which public programs will turn to to provide the supplementary help needed, or what manpower the family will turn to.

Selma Fraiberg,[8] speaking mainly of children, points out that what children need primarily is "mothering," that is, physical contact in care, a person who will respond to attempts at communication and will help fulfill the need for bodily care and physical and emotional security. Although adults who are severely disabled may not need anything called "mothering," they do need other individuals who provide physical contact, who maintain communication—at least share in providing food and bodily care and physical security. This need is requisite even for the young adult with the spinal cord injury who has been fully "rehabilitated" and is able to go out and hold a remunerative job—such a person requires attendant care some part of the day from others for the procurement of minimum mobility and minimum physical security. But for the vulnerable population of which we are speaking, who will provide this "mothering"? With the labor force as demanding of family manpower as it seems to be, it appears that our only option would be to industrialize the caring function, that is, to organize corporations and agencies which will hire people out of families to go back into other families to provide caring. Whether this kind of industrialization of a labor-intensive function can be carried out at a reasonable economic level remains to be seen. But if we are to in fact be a caring society, it's going to be necessary to take some such approach and to provide incomes to the industrialized workers who provide the caring at an acceptable and attractive competitive wage.

4. Another possibility, perhaps strange to our ears, might be

called the *quid pro quo* policy. A. R. Hands[9] reports the original concept of philanthropy in ancient Greece was one of reciprocity, deriving from exchanges of friendship between status equals. When an individual needed or desired something, he turned to a status equal who gave this to him, and this in turn obligated the beneficiary to act in like fashion to the benefactor. Over time, even in ancient Greece, this concept of reciprocity was ultimately extended to include benefits given from a higher status to a lower status person, but it was still expected that the individual of lower status responded in some fashion reciprocally, even if it was only by voting honors and benefits to the grantor in the nature of praise and the like. Under such a reciprocal policy, one might, in a crude fashion, articulate it somewhat as follows: (a) if you are working and pay taxes and you have a troubled family member, the state will help you if you contribute to the cost; (b) if you don't work, the state will help you but you have to do some part of the caring with your own labor, too. It is possible, under such a reciprocal scheme, to use money and the time necessary to provide help as some kind of reasonable measure about what is to be expected from family members as part of the reciprocal scheme.

We are accustomed to think of measurements in an industrial society primarily in terms of dollars, but it is possible that when we speak about family relationships and family responsibilities vis-à-vis the state, we might be better advised to turn to some less economic measure such as time (which, of course, does have an economic value). Is it possible to argue that there is some volume of time, apart from its monetary value, which all family members can be expected to devote to the care of other vulnerable members of that family? When the amount of time required by the recipient exceeds this "reasonable measure," this could become the trigger mechanism by which public supplements are introduced to work much like a deductible does in an insurance policy.

Some clues about this are already available. The Urban Institute[10] estimates for example that when personal care is needed up to 10 hours a day it can be met by many alternatives, including family care: over 10 hours *a day* clearly calls for institutional care. Eggert, Morris et al.[11] found that in a sample of chronically ill patients cared for by their families over a 6-month period of time, an average of 12 hours of care at home per week sufficed to continue home care and could be tolerated by family members.

Between such extremes a reasonable measure of time burden on families could be located. Needs identified above this threshold would be met by some social program, up to a maximum to be specified—health insurance, a social service, etc. In such an approach, the first unit of effort or money is provided by the family as a deductible; beyond that, some social supplement is triggered. Alternatively, one could argue that this minimum should be just guaranteed by a social provision for all and that more generous care then is provided by family or friends. The poor probably fare better under this latter approach in which the first dollar spent is public.

## A FINAL ORGANIZATIONAL NOTE

Such broad brush policy choices each require some organizational skeleton by which they can be structured operationally and their aims be realized. Sketchily, these are some possibilities.

1. *A demogrant or an aid and attendance allowance* for the person who is disabled, be he old or young, is attractive and least complicated. Under it, vulnerable persons are classified by their disability level in much the same way that we now identify for SSI or insurance eligibility. We have precedents for this. The United Kingdom has had for some time a disability attendance allowance which is payable to an individual found by expert judgment to need the attention of another adult some time during the day or the night. The allowance is a flat sum, payable to the individual regardless of other sources of income. It is not a sum intended to meet all the needs that the individual may have. The individual is still expected to do much for himself, or his family or neighbors are expected to do much, but the allowance is a public recognition that human attention must be secured beyond normal income replacement or family help for persons who are severely disabled. The sums paid are a maximum of $31.20 (1978 exchange rate) per week, payable regardless of what other social benefits are available, although nominal payment for use of other benefits is expected. About 57% of the beneficiaries are aged, 17% are other adults including the adult retarded, and 15% are children, many also retarded.

In the U.S. we have precedent for the same system in the Veterans Administration, which identifies and classifies veterans according to disability incurred in the military service, and makes cash payments to them according to the level of their disability.

Such an allowance is a cash payment in addition to normal income replacement, such as that provided by Supplementary Security Income, it recognizes the disability increment or deficit, and involves some expansion in public expenditure, but such an allowance would be offset in part as it replaces some expenditure now fruitlessly misplaced on curative efforts which cannot cure, or as it offsets payments now being made through a variety of separate channels such as Title XX to the Social Security Act, the Rehabilitation Services Administration, and a community mental health system. Such a system also requires expert screening and assessment, but the authority of expert judgment does not go beyond the identification of an existing condition which requires a personal attendant some of the time. Once that is done, the individuals are free to use the supplement or the disability allowance in any way they individually see fit.

(Such a program would not remove the necessity for some safety net for what I believe to be a relatively small percentage of persons who would be so incapable of functioning that more extensive responsibility would have to be taken for them. Into this category might fall some proportion of children for whom the total burden on the family is so great that the family collapses or is in danger of collapsing and perhaps those adults lacking family supports who are found legally to be incompetent to manage their own affairs. This is not the place to discuss the complexity of and the limitations of a possible safety net, but I would like to only note that such a safety net provision probably is necessary regardless of the general policy finally adopted.)

2. Some form of *social insurance* for the long-term disabled, in addition to insurance for acute medical care, could be considered. This differs from a demogrant in that risk sharing includes some premium payment by covered persons. Nursing home and home health care are now insured, in a minimum way, through Medicare and some private companies. Such insurance could be expanded by increasing the duration of home health and nursing home benefits, by making access to home care benefits more flexible, and by adding coverage for personal care services above home medical treatment. Being a cash program the organizational mechanisms are partly in place, but these have had no experience with payments for non-medical services which would have to be added, and the control of which may be difficult. The scope of new demand and utilization that would be released is not well

known, since we do not know whether families, which now give 80% of personal care without compensation, would continue to do so or would shift the cost to insurance reimbursement.

3. One promising approach which still needs to be tested empirically might be called a *Social and Health Maintenance Organization*.[12] Such an organization can be organized under medical, welfare, or other auspices. An S/HMO would have the following characteristics: (a) responsibility for an enrolled or specified population which can be handled either on the basis of enrollment or geographical assignment; (b) a staff consisting of both professional health and non-professional caring personnel; (c) provides a range of services to the enrolled population which spans physical and social care at home through ambulatory medical and social treatment to institutional care; (d) payment from a third party or by premiums based on capitation, meaning an annual sum for enrolled members sufficient to cover the range of guaranteed services expected to be used by the population covered, but assuming that not all people require all services at the same time. Such an organization then retains within its own staff the responsibility for deciding the best distribution of services and the distribution of resources, but is in sufficiently close contact with its beneficiary population to be more responsive to individual variation than are regulations embedded in law and requiring long periods of time to change. There are risks of reduced quality care inherent in any capitation scheme.

4. *A single unified long-term care program* can be fully visualized. There is a certain logic for arguing that persons who are vulnerable all require certain common care which may be more important than their differences; such as, attention to communication, mobility, physical needs, etc.

A single program could be organized as a generic funding device, consolidating some parts of Medicaid, Title XX social services, Rehabilitation Services, Community Mental Health, and of the Administration on Aging. Consolidated funding would transfer decision power from the Congress to an executive administration to chose resource allocation and the service delivery channels to use. It would not, of itself, solve any of the current problems of underfunding or of discontinuity in services. Some argue that there would be administrative savings and greater efficiencies, but the evidence about economies flowing from large scale organization are not compelling in the human services field.

A single program could also be organized around service delivery, not funding. Such a structure has been anticipated in the Kennedy Corman Health Insurance Bill which calls for a network of disability assessment centers to judge levels of need and to arrange for care accordingly. However, there has not been tested at the delivery of services level a program which would provide all necessary services under one administration for all the disabled—the developmentally disabled child, the aged, the work injured adult, etc.—so our ability to manage limited resources better under a single administration than under specialized ones remains a theory, not a proven means. The S/HMO suggested above is one form of consolidation.

5. It is possible to visualize *keeping our categorical programs* for each major age-defined or condition-defined condition, but making each one more comprehensive than is now the case. There is no reason for believing that a program which concentrates, let us say, solely on neurologically damaged children must concentrate its effort solely upon rehabilitation, cure, or medical attention while ignoring the social caring and physical caring responsibilities we have been talking about. Whether there is one generic program or several remains a matter of choice which needs further experimentation and political debate.

There is much to be said for incrementally improving our existing structures rather than trying out brave and major reorganizations which lack clear evidence as to their likely results. In only 13 years we have erected an extensive array of caring programs. We cover much medical and nursing home care for the poor and disabled as well as for the well-to-do and episodically ill; we have recently expanded our options for care by significantly increasing home care agencies and funding for their support; and Congress this year finally authorized extension of rehabilitation services of many kinds, including attendant care, to increase opportunities for self-care as well as for work. While the resource distribution among these parts is still askew and while there are discontinuities among them, it is possible that the deficiencies in our present categorical system are minor when compared with the rapid advances of recent years. If it were to turn out, on close examination, that present defects flaw only 20% of the system or of the population in need we may be able to improve that marginal 20% by improving each category faster and more efficiently than by trying to dismantle the present system and replace it with an untested new model. At least such a heretical notion should not be rejected out of hand.

After this discursive foray into policy choices, it must remain clear that the doubts and uncertainties perhaps overwhelm the few bases for moving ahead.

There is no one option which is overwhelmingly better than all others. At best each has advantages and disadvantages so that we must make our trade-offs by debate and by political preference. We *can* make the trade-offs more clear.

What we need is a common screen against which we can judge each option. Until we have such a screen we can only crudely note such aspects as these: any program of cash to the individual will increase patient power in decision making, but we do not know if that will be strong enough to alter the behavior of professional providers or the supply of varied services. On the other hand, publicly funded programs shift the decision center from the patient to the provider who is funded. Either a cash or a service program can bias its benefits or incentives to favor the poor or the middle class, to favor the most disabled or the least, or to transfer more or less uncompensated family effort to public funding. A locally administered program will probably be more restrictive if past history is any guide, and it will result in more variety and unevenness in benefits across the nation than any nationally administered program, but the local decision making keeps freedom of choice closer to our informal social structure.

One thing remains clear to me. We are going through a period of grave uncertainty in the field of social welfare and social policy. Uncertainties and doubts about our trust in the state have become corrosive. At the same time, the very civilizing tendencies of all history require that we not abandon the caring function which has been so painstakingly elaborated over the decades. We are in an era when we are struggling somehow to maintain this civilizing caring sense while at the same time not abdicating entirely to a faceless and anonymous state. Just how we will walk this tightrope depends upon our convictions and sense of confidence. I see no hope for a reasonable solution that relies entirely upon the individual. The major hope that does derive from a discussion about the American family lies in the fact that it does talk about a collective entity known as the family and, by extension, the collective responsibility which all families constituting a society ultimately have for their own future. How we strike the balance between individual realization and our sense of responsibility to each other will decide the character and livability or worthwhileness of the world in which we live.

## REFERENCES

1. See, for example, Willard Gaylin, Ira Glasser, Steven Marcus, and David Rothman, *Doing Good, The Limits of Benevolence.* New York: Pantheon Books, 1978; Maurice Janowitz, *Social Control of the Welfare State.* Chicago: University of Chicago Press, 1976; Kathleen Nott, *The Good Want Power*: and many others.

2. W. Gaylin, J. Glasser, S. Marcus, D. Rothman, *Doing Good—The Limits of Benevolence, Pantheon, N.Y., 1978*; M. Janowitz, *Social Control of the Welfare State,* U. of Chicago Press, Chicago, 1976.

3. Louis Harris & Assoc./National Council on Aging, "The Myth and Realities of Aging in American." See also, Mary Jo Bane, *Here to Stay: American Families in the 20th Century,* New York: Basic Books.

4. See Harris Poll, *op. cit.*; and G. Bultena, "Rural-Urban Differences in the Familial Interaction of the Aged," *Rural Sociology,* 1969, Vol. 34; and Shanas and others, *Old People in Three Industrial Societies,* New York: Atherton Press; and Kevin J. Mahoney, *A National Perspective on Community Differences in the Interaction of the Aged with their Adult Children,* the Faye-McBeath Institute, University of Wisconsin, Madison (mimeo).

5. Kirsten Gronbjerg, *Mass Society and the Extension of Welfare,* University of Chicago Press, 1977.

6. See T. H. Marshall, *Class, Citizenship and Social Development,* Garden City, N.Y.: Doubleday Press, 1964.

7. Murray Edelman, *Political Language,* Academic Press, Inc., 1977.

8. Selma Fraiberg, *Every Child's Birthright: In Defense of Mothering.* New York; Basic Books.

9. A. R. Hands, *Charities and Social Aid in Greece and Rome.* London: Thames & Hudson, 1968.

10. "Final Report, Study of Federal Policies Related to the Disabled." Urban Institute, Aug. 1975, Washington, D.C.

11. Gerald Eggert et al. "Community Based Maintenance Care for the Long-term Patient." Levinson Policy Institute, Brandeis University, 1976.

12. In 1981-82 the University Health Policy Consortium, Brandeis University, began a field test of this approach with support from the Health Care Finance Administration and several regional foundations.

# Designs for Home-Care Entitlements

Dwight L. Frankfather
Michael J. Smith
Francis G. Caro

As the United States moves toward a home-care entitlement for the chronically disabled, major policy questions remain unsolved. The FSP* has provided an opportunity to probe these questions while emphasizing the relationships between the family and the state. Family assumption of home-care responsibility is so widespread that it must be considered a crucial factor in the development of long-term care policy. Yet decisions regarding the role of the family and the extent of its responsibility have not obtained the visibility and consideration they deserve. Furthermore, credible objectives, realistic standards, and plausible program designs have not been clearly conceptualized for the long-term care field in general. The process of planning and evaluating the FSP has made clear the limitations of conventional wisdom in this field. Therefore alternative formulations for design objectives and standards are recommended in the concluding two chapters.

## *TWO-TIER ENTITLEMENT*

The FSP is important as a demonstration because the two-tier entitlement policy may have appeal to federal policymakers; thus its feasibility must be evaluated carefully. One tier would provide complete personal maintenance care for impaired elderly without family support. For those with families, the second tier would provide very modest benefits to complement but not replace family contributions. The experience with FSP suggests that such a policy merits consideration. The project had no difficulty in locating fam-

Reprinted by permission of the publisher, from FAMILY CARE OF THE ELDERLY by Dwight L. Frankfather, Michael J. Smith, and Francis G. Caro (Lexington, Mass.: Lexington Books, D. C. Heath and Company).

*The Family Support Program of the Community Service Society of New York.

ilies who were assuming substantial responsibility for an impaired older adult. In fact, a large number of inquiries were received after very little publicity about the program. The service applicants wanted to continue their role and welcomed help. Relatives expressed deep personal obligations to disabled elderly members and dreaded the specter of institutionalization. Families experienced severe restrictions and regimentation in life-style that made them desperate for assistance.

The impaired person and other family members generally did not object to open discussion of service needs at a family meeting that the staff organized. In fact, the family members appreciated the opportunity. There were instances, however, in which the family members could not agree among themselves about service needs. At times, supporting members disagreed with each other and objected to the disabled person's preferences. Unfortunately the FSP model does not prescribe any standard solution to such dilemmas other than withholding benefits until a consensus is reached. The problem resides in treating the family as the eligible unit. It can be argued, however, that any program design would encounter potential users who objected to procedures or refused assistance. In spite of this limitation, the programmatic concept clearly establishes relief of family as a legitimate social objective. Relief is granted, however, only if the family accepts the terms of the offer and the authority of the provider to determine benefits.

The staff was able to negotiate modest service levels with family members, sustain their participation, and avoid escalation of demands. Faced with uncertainty about available service options and about benefit limitations, family members acquiesced to provider instruction. The homemaker service unquestionably was useful to family members, as well as to the disabled person. Family members claimed that the introduction of service helped them sustain their efforts. Family members did understand and agree to continue their support as a condition of eligibility. It appears, therefore, that modest benefits reduce the disincentive effect that results from a more-generous program for those without family resources. It is important for benefits to be attractive enough to minimize the artificial dissolution of family ties so that older disabled persons can qualify for higher benefit levels available to those without family resources. It is hoped that family support benefits could be structured so that public costs would be manageable. If successful, the two-tier strategy should substantially reduce the aggregate cost of a home-care entitlement. A cost-suppression effect is the strongest argument in favor of the plan.

The prominence of the family variable, however, conceptually weakens the social basis for a home-care entitlement and leads to serious operational flaws. There is a public responsibility to provide an adequate and humane level of existence for those who must cope with serious and unalterable impairments. Therefore it is reasonable to defray the costs of their care among the members of society at large. Receipt of benefits is conditioned upon the presence of serious disabilities in the same way that Medicare and Medicaid provide benefits for the eligible who suffer illness or injury. It is contradictory to argue for a disability-based entitlement and simultaneously to assert that families must assume principal responsibility. There is a risk that the contradiction would lead to a confusion of purpose in a national program.

In the United States, social insurance programs are much more palatable to the electorate than are public assistance and welfare. For this reason, it would be desirable if long-term care programs adhered as closely as possible to an insurance model of testing eligibility and setting benefits. An insurance model further emphasizes the direct disability-benefit relationship. Again, it would be difficult to argue that chronic disability insurance benefits would be paid only if family support was absent. For instance Medicare, a comparable insurance plan, pays health-care costs of the elderly regardless of the presence or absence of family capacity.

In addition to the problems created by the conceptual confusion and contradictions inherent in the two-tier plan, there would be obstacles in implementation. Determining the presence or absence of family is not necessarily simple. Clearly a disabled older adult without known living relatives could be categorized as being without family, but other conditions are more difficult to define. The issue is not mere presence but the degree of capacity to provide, as well as the legal obligation to do so. Measures of family capacity might include the number of relatives, their geographic proximity, their competence, their frailty or disability, their willingness, the quality of their relationship with the impaired member, and the extent of their other occupational and familial responsibilities. This collection of variables cannot readily be summed up into a uniform measure of family capacity and obligation.

The inevitable inconsistencies can be demonstrated through examples from FSP cases. Since adult daughters frequently are the primary supporting relative, presumably eligibility decisions would be based in part on their role. Would an adult daughter living a thousand miles away be held as responsible as well as one living ten miles away? Would the required degree of responsibility be proportional to their geographic distance? What would be the proportions? Would the contribution required of a retired adult daughter be greater than of an employed adult daughter? Or should a lesser contribution be expected of the more-aged daughter? Would an adult daughter without child-care duties be required to accept greater responsibility than one with young children to care for? Would the numbers, health, and age of children be considered? Should the adult daughter who suffers ill health or disability be required to make a smaller contribution than one who is healthy? Should the health and abilities of the adult daughter's husband be considered?

A fully operationalized two-tier plan would need to assess each legally responsible relative, including the spouse, siblings, and other adult children, on these variables. Which of these relatives could in fact be held legally responsible when many states no longer even hold spouses responsible for the costs of nursing-home care?

Family members in FSP did not always agree among themselves about who should do what or how much. Sometimes they disagreed with the disabled person about service needs. Under such conditions, would the state choose among the responsible relatives and assign responsibilities?

It remains to be shown that family contributions could actually be enforced. Would family members sever their ties rather than tolerate imposed obligations they considered unreasonable? When the disabled person or a primary supporting family member moved away, would a shift to a more-generous benefit tier automatically follow? Would it be necessary to uncover the motivation for relocation? If family members were caught evading responsibilities would they be penalized?

Attempts to measure and enforce family contributions would result in enormous inconsistencies and inequities. There would be no standardization in the distribution of benefits. Obviously the costs of collecting such a large volume of data on every applicant's family would be prohibitive. The unstructured case assessment and monitoring style employed in FSP was also expensive. And it would be vulnerable to wide benefit variations among programs and among staff within programs. If an ill-conceived and operationally flawed national entitlement design is the best that can be accomplished in an era of retrenching social services, then inaction and delay may be preferable to expansion.

## A MAINTENANCE-MODEL APPROACH

How should a home-care entitlement and a nationwide service industry be structured? Whether or not a two-tier design is adopted in the future, the question is pertinent. The FSP data do provide an empirical basis for anticipating operational obstacles in program designs similar to FSP and for recommending alternative solutions. Recruitment and eligibility, benefit levels, domain of covered services, management, cost control, and impact on beneficiaries are the basic components of public programs. The pieces must be assembled in a way that is functionally practical and internally coherent while meeting basic performance criteria for public sector programs. There is general consensus that public benefits should be equitably distributed, services should be of high quality, management should be efficient, and cost should be controllable. To some extent, these desirable characteristics must be balanced and compromised. For example, a program with intense service monitoring might produce high-quality care, but the administrative costs might be unacceptably high. A well-conceived program inevitably requires a sophisticated and delicately structured package.

In contrast to the professional model, which tends to be characteristic of community-based, long-term care demonstrations, is a maintenance model. The model emphasizes user control of benefits and standardized determinations of eligibility and benefit level. It also relies more heavily on market incentives to control quality and production costs. The principles of diagnosis, etiology, treatment, and rehabilitation that characterize the professional model are only marginally relevant to the maintenance of the chronically disabled. The purpose of home care here is to maintain, not to rehabilitate. Rather than placing responsibility for determining need, level of benefit utilization, prescription, delivery and case management in the hands of one professional, the functions are segregated and independently regulated in the maintenance model.

### Recruitment and Eligibility

In federal public entitlement programs such as food stamps, social security, Medicare, and Medicaid a premium is placed on the equitable distribution of benefits. Theoretically, uniform and consistent treatment of applications results in similar benefits for persons with similar characteristics and in similar circumstances. This principle is highly valued in the United States and rests on a constitutional commitment to equal treatment under the law. A serious commitment to equitable distribution of home-care benefits to the chronically impaired would be operationalized with recruitment plans that resulted in high application rates from potential beneficiaries and standardized and consistent assessments of eligibility. The maintenance model would require strict disability testing to determine eligibility. The presence, absence, or degree of functional impairment is measured, and eligibility and benefit-level decisions are based on predetermined standards. Standards would be set so that only the seriously and chronically impaired received service.

In some states, variations of disability tests are practiced in the form of nursing-home preadmission screening and assessment instruments for community-care programs. Many of these instruments are constructed however, so that functional impairment and disagnostic information are interwoven. Usually such instruments are identified as psychosocial assessment. They include not only impairment data but also information on the respondent's degree of cheerfulness, happiness, anxiety, agitation, gregariousness, and personal satisfaction with life. The assessment instrument becomes cluttered with variables, many of them inappropriate for disability testing. Lack of cheerfulness and gregariousness are personality traits, not indicators of functional impairment. It is doubtful that they should be among eligibility criteria for public programs.

Even when dimensions of impairment are valid, the indicators of performance are often ambiguous and subject to interviewer interpretation. For example, disability items are sometimes scaled as follows: "performs task adequately with no assistance," "performs adequately with assistance," "performs tasks adequately with occasional assistance," and so forth. The key words are *adequate, assistance,* and *occasional.* Consider a task like bathing. What is "adequate" bathing? Is the ability to take a thorough sponge bath independently at the sink adequate bathing? If it is considered inadequate, should it be equated with the inability to bathe at all? What does *assistance* mean? Is that a handrail or bathtub bar? Or is that an attendant who physically lifts the impaired person from the tub? If they are both forms of assistance, should they be equated? Finally, how often is occasional? Is it once a day or once a week? Does the meaning of the word occasional vary with the task? The use of words like *adequate, assistance,* and *occasional* leaves much opportunity for individual interpretation. Most, but not all, of that interpretation can be removed when concrete indicators replace personal judgment. Accomplishing this is not a serious methodological problem.

The means of administering the instrument is probably more important than the instrument itself. Consistent use of a measurement tool requires training. As the number of assessors increases, the error due to inconsistent interpretation inevitably increases. There is a risk of random inconsistencies in measurement. Therefore it is desirable to minimize the number of people administering the disability test. Perhaps more important than random error, however, is the risk of systematic distortion (or instrument corruption), which can result when the party administering the measurement has vested interests to protect. For instance, in nursing-home preadmission screening, the level of care available often dictates the score rather than the score determining the level of care. Any measurement tool would be seriously corrupted if it were administered by the service provider (or even the case manager) who had responsibility for a recipient's level of benefits and therefore, the quality of care. The burden of securing care and the burden of withholding benefits cannot be given to the same person without resulting in measurement distortion and inconsistency.

With adjustments in present instruments and administration of assessments, disability measurement is an attractive basis for distributing benefits equitably. But the instrument should be very concrete and consist of a small and manageable number of dimensions. Furthermore, control over the administration of the test must remain organizationally independent of the service-delivery and case-management components. Eligibility specialists should be trained and directly employed by the government. This quite conventional idea is comparable to the separation of eligibility from service in welfare progams today.

### Take-up Rates

The take-up rate is the percentage of apparently eligible persons in the population who apply for and receive entitled benefits. The application rate for a national home-care entitlement program could be somewhere between 25 and 95 percent of the eligibles. Variable take-up rates have profound cost implications. In a cost-conscious service era, a low take-up rate could appear attractive. The take-up rate can be readily manipulated. The existence of long waiting lists, lengthy turnaround times on application decisions, extensive documentation requirements, retroactive denials, frequent recertifications, and a demeaning manner among eligibility workers will help to discourage applicants from enduring the eligibility process. If home-care programs can be administered without such informal, discretionary controls, they offer more promise as an institutional alternative. If services were in adequate supply, available promptly, and considered to be reliable and attractive by beneficiaries, hospital discharge staff, physicians in private practice, and others, home care would become a more credible alternative. For the sake of consistency and equitability in the distribution of benefits through public bureaucracies, home-care programs should be designed to encourage high take-up rates. For the sake of predicting and containing expenditures, eligibility should be regulated with strict and explicit criteria.

To attract potential applicants, entitlement benefits and eligibility criteria should be widely advertised in the mass media. Extensive and detailed information should be printed in brochures and widely distributed. Announcements should be carefully worded to include a list of covered services, a thorough description of disability-testing and benefit-reduction criteria, and instructions for making application.

## *Benefit Levels and Benefit Reductions*

A maintenance model would also promise more-generous benefits to those with greater functional impairment. The principle of uniform treatment would be satisfied by setting predetermined capitation rates. The cash value of the benefit would be indexed to the level of disability. The degree of precision in scaling benefits would be determined by the best precision obtainable in a disability instrument that gave consistent results. The actual cash values would be determined by the political process. They would reflect the willingness of the electorate to pay for the maintenance of the disabled. Assigning a predetermined benefit on the basis of a disability score is a mundane chore for a functionary.

Predetermined benefit rates might be reduced by a fixed formula that takes into account the applicant's ability to pay (means test) and the capacity of the family to provide support. There are precedents for both inclusion and omission of means testing in public entitlements. Means tests are characteristic of the welfare programs but not insurance programs. It would be desirable for reasons of operational efficiency and public tolerance to structure home-care entitlement as an insurance rather than a welfare program.

Means tests typically measure assets and income. Experience with asset testing in nursing-home placement suggests it may be impractical. Pauperization is a politically explosive topic. It has been very difficult to detect or prevent asset transfers to family members. It is not clear that asset-related revenues have been worth the political and administrative trouble they cause. If income testing is introduced into a maintenance model, it should be done in a palatable way. In a disability program in which the cash value of the benefits is predetermined and fixed according to the level of disability, income above a maximum limit could result in a proportional benefit reduction rather than a loss of eligibility. Of course, this is comparable to the Social Security Administration's approach to income testing, which is required for all those eligible under the age of seventy-two. Although this model deviates from traditional Medicaid and welfare income tests, there are no inherent obstacles to the benefit-reduction model in a disability program with fixed capitation rates, and politically, it is more agreeable to users and to the aging constituency at large.

Family capacity has too many dimensions to permit testing for eligibility purposes. Furthermore, the norm of obligatory family contributions would also need to be defined. If there is some limit to the extent of family responsibility, how will it be measured and specified? Standardized assessments and norms appear unrealistic.

### Covered Services

A maintenance model for a home-care entitlement would not promise all covered services to all beneficiaries. It would promise the opportunity to select from among covered services up to the cash-value limit on the benefit level. In FSP, families routinely either sought or provided a variety of services:

—Homemaker services, including cooking, shopping, house-cleaning, and laundry.

—Personal care services, including bathing, toileting, feeding, exercise, medication, assistance in walking, and companionship.
—Prosthetic equipment and other supplies that contribute to the safety and independence of the impaired client.
—Heavy-duty housecleaning and home maintenance that is beyond the capacity of the impaired client but periodically required.
—Transportation, including only the use of conventionally equipped automobiles, taxis, and public transportation without restriction on destination.
—Assistance with entitlements, including information and referal, and case monitoring.
—Telephone security checks to ensure that a client's unanticipated illness, accident, or injury does not go unnoticed.
—Assistance with personal bookkeeping and financial management.
—Location of adequate shelter and the means necessary to accomplish relocation.
—Case management.

This list constitutes an inclusive but defined domain of care for the maintenance of the chronically disabled. Medical and health specialty services provided under existing entitlements—physician care, skilled nursing, skilled therapies, and counseling—have not been included.

### Benefit Payments and Case Accounts

In the maintenance model, services are claimed by users rather than assigned by experts. To ensure beneficiary control over selection, the cash value or benefits would be paid directly to the user. A benefit account would be opened with the public agency responsible for administering the entitlement, and beneficiaries would draw from their accounts for the purchase of the covered services they choose. The process for handling claims and reimbursement sometimes is defined as a voucher mechanism. The principle is similar to the administration of the food stamp program.

Once benefit levels were established by the government, professional expertise would not be required to diagnose the need to have floors scrubbed, windows washed, linen laundered, warm meals prepared, and so forth. In many instances the need for such items reflects the beneficiaries' personal preferences. This argument is reinforced by the failure of experts to agree with one another in diagnosing the home-care needs of a particular case.[1] In FSP, there were notable discrepancies between user preferences and professional prescription. Assistance in shopping for home-care options among suppliers will be required by some or many disabled persons, but this function is not equivalent to diagnosis and prescription. Some users might desire comprehensive case management, and they would be able to purchase it, like any other covered service, from their benefit account.

Public confidence in the feasibility of home care rests in part on sound evidence that public money will be spent for the designated purposes and the products will be of reasonable quality. A case accountant role is necessary to provide public accountability for benefit expenditures. In the professional model, this function is one of many assumed by a case manager. For this reason, the term *case accountant* is preferred even though it may imply a narrower range of responsibilities than is intended. The case accountant would offer advice and information on where the desired services could be obtained and on the relative merits and costs of the various options. Case accountants would review claims on their clients' accounts. Claims could be made by local suppliers of covered service and equipment, by beneficiaries, and by individuals employed by beneficiaries to provide covered services. Case accountants would also monitor the quality of direct service. Management and counseling functions would be segregated. In the professional model, a home visit every other week may be good counseling, but this convention should not dictate monitoring procedures. Counseling is a treatment strategy. If it were a covered service, it would be purchased out of the benefit account.

The nature of the relationship between the case accountant and the user makes the line between advice and coercion potentially vague. The influence of case accountants will be great in cases when a severely disabled user has no family or agent other than the accountant. Therefore when service claims are substantially altered or benefits denied for any reason other than exclusion by regulation, some formalized denial-of-service procedure should be required. In addition, beneficiaries should have a mechanism by which they can initiate a review of denials. (Similar review procedures should exist for disability testing and other eligibility criteria.) Beneficiaries who find it difficult to work with one case accountant should have the opportunity to switch to another. The maintenance model presumes that functionally impaired individuals are neither mentally incompetent nor pathologically irrational. The presumption will not hold true in every case. Beneficiaries may also be victimized by manipulative caretakers who do not act in their best interests. Reasonable case accountants and users may also simply disagree on interpretation of regulations. To some extent, disagreements can be expected as part of normal routine and are not indicative of program failure. In this model, the burden of proof for the right to deny service would rest with the agent of the state, presumably the case accountant.

## Suppliers of Service and Equipment

In the maintenance model, users would be free to choose their own providers. It would be desirable for beneficiaries to have multiple sources of service from which to choose. Among the regular choices would be not-for-profit organizations, voluntary agencies, for-profit agencies, and self-recruited personnel, including relatives, neighbors, and friends. Whenever one sector of the service industry is being expanded, considerable debate follows over the designation of eligible providers. The competing providers seek to capture as much of the future service dollars as possible by claiming a superior service capacity; their income, jobs, profit, and prestige are at stake. The for-profit agencies claim efficiency and dependability. Their detractors claim that the profit motive leads to skimpy services and that the quality of care is subject to deterioration. The voluntary agencies claim high professional standards and objectivity in assessing need. Their competitors claim that administrative inefficiency and unnecessarily enriched service packages lead to unnecessarily high costs. Clients may be attracted by the reduced costs of employing an independent homemaker or attendant at minimum wage and avoiding all administrative costs. This might lead, however, to the employment of unqualified persons and might prove to be costly and cumbersome for a public agency to administer. Clients may prefer to "hire" family members and thus avoid opening their homes to strangers or being subjected to personal and intimate handling by unknown persons. Opponents to this practice argue that it is difficult to monitor cash flows and ensure that the designated services are actually provided. No clear advantage in quality of care belongs to any single source of service. For this reason, competition among all of them would be encouraged. Ideally producers would seek to attract beneficiaries with imaginative service packages and low fees.

It is clear from the FSP data that the nature of services obtainable from existing homemaker agencies is in need of great improvement. There were frequent problems with homemaker reliability and compatibility with the user. Home care could not be purchased for short, irregular periods or before 9:00 A.M. and after 5:00 P.M. A combination of housecleaning and personal care was difficult to find, and the fee was considerably higher than for housecleaning alone. There was no twenty-four-hour-a-day intervention capacity for emergencies. With such extensive limitations and flaws, homemaker agencies could not provide a credible alternative to institutional care, regardless of the level of funding that might be available. In either a professional or maintenance model, a more-sophisticated delivery organization is required. Undoubtedly it would be necessary for public agencies to define the required delivery capacity and to stimulate the formation of suitable provider organizations.[2]

In FSP, the employment of independent operators, including relatives and friends, yielded a generally high level of service. The flexibility and reliability of relatives, neighbors, and friends exceeded that obtainable from agencies. Presumably fees for independent operators with no overhead would be less than organizational reimbursement rates. Impaired elderly with families willing to supervise independent operators could absorb some administrative costs and obtain more direct service for each benefit dollar.

The suggestion that relatives, particularly a spouse, be allowed reimbursement at a reasonable rate for their services usually invites skepticism and sometimes alarm. Nonetheless, in a disability-based entitlement program, the exclusion of family members from reimbursement is difficult to defend. In a few FSP cases, a spouse or adult child was near retirement and might have preferred reimbursable home care as substitute employment. Judging from FSP data, concern over quality of care is more of an incentive than an obstacle for reimbursing family members.

## Control of Case Management and Administrative Costs

Personnel salaries are the principal source of costs for home care. Personnel can be divided into two levels: direct production, and management and administration. Regarding direct production, the cost of employing a homemaker or a personal attendant is basically a matter of salary and benefits. Degrees of investment in fringe benefits, training, equipment, supplies, uniforms, and transportation will produce some variation in direct cost. The nature of the variables does make them subject to government standard setting, monitoring, and regulation. That is the easier part of cost control.

Unlike the direct costs, case management and other administrative costs will vary enormously and will be more difficult to regulate. It may be that 40 to 50 percent of a home-care agency's costs ultimately will be attributable to administrative expenses. For example, the Community Care Organization of Milwaukee County reported that indirect costs were 39 percent of total expenditures.[3] In FSP, indirect costs ranged between 50 and 60 percent of total expenditures. The final report for Triage, a Medicare-financed home-care demonstration, showed that over 50 percent of the expenditures were for indirect costs.[4] In one highly professionalized home-care demonstration project in Chicago, homemaker services are reimbursed at a rate of $12 per hour. Of this $12, only 40 percent ($4.75) is attributable to homemaker salary. The remaining 60 percent covers administrative costs, excluding bookkeeping, which is donated by a local hospital. Each of these illustrations leads to the regrettable conclusion that an administrative cost rate of only 50 percent might be the best that can be achieved in these programs. But is it reasonable to spend forty to fifty cents out of every home-care dollar on administration at the project level, to say nothing about the expenses attributable to state or federal responsibilities for management?

In comparison to the professional model, there are potential administrative cost savings in the maintenance model. Since an eligibility specialist with a single, straightforward disability test could replace diagnostically oriented assessments by professionals, nearly the same purpose would be accomplished in less time and at a lower cost. The service-assignment function usually claimed by professionals would be assumed by beneficiaries who shopped

among suppliers for home care. Those unable to shop for themselves would require assistance. A clear distinction between management and counseling would permit less-intrusive and less-expensive monitoring procedures. Presumably a reduction and a
deprofessionalization of the middle-man role will reduce administrative costs.[5]

Many of the cost-control strategies adopted for nursing-home reimbursement may be applicable to home care. In the coming years,
there may be rate ceilings, single invoicing, regulated profit factors, limitation on pass throughs, indexing, fee schedules, utilization limitations, rate reviews, recovery programs for third-party
liability, and certificates of need for home care. These strategies
have not always been as successful as expected in regulating nursing-home care. Taking greater advantage of market incentives
in a disability program, however, could complement regulatory
activities and perhaps reduce reliance on cost-control regulations
altogether.

## SUMMARY

Attempts to measure, define norms, and enforce family contributions to maintenance of seriously impaired elderly would lead to
inconsistent and inequitable distributions of public benefits. A two-
tier design is unlikely to satisfy minimum performance criteria for
public programs. Nonetheless families do respond to incentives
and generally are willing to work with external actors on problems
in providing care. Therefore a disability-based public-entitlement
program that openly acknowledged and rewarded family support
might be the best solution.

It might also be the most expensive solution. If there was explicit and full assumption of public responsibility in a disability-
insurance model, it is unlikely that family members would continue to provide care without making the claims for reimbursement
to which they were entitled. To control costs, disability-based
eligibility criteria would need to be simple, explicit, and strin-
gently enforced. Also disability entrance standards would need
to be high. Only the seriously disabled would obtain access to
benefits.

Middle-level management would be nonintrusive. With predetermined capitation rates and strict disability testing, benefit levels
would be efficiently and economically determined. Counseling

functions would not overlap with case monitoring. Case accountants would provide public accountability and assistance to users. Suppliers might be independent operators, existing homemaker agencies, or new organizations that can provide an expanded range of benefits. Beneficiaries would have authority to select from a clearly specified domain of covered services and choose the provider that they prefer. Measurement of quality would focus on actual service delivery rather than the licensing of providers.

Overall cost control would rely chiefly on regulation of demand for care. Authority to test disability and benefit levels would remain the prerogative of the state. Administrative costs would be minimized by reducing management authority and the extent of supervision and counseling of users. Entrepreneurial service suppliers would be encouraged to compete with existing agencies and independent operators. Suppliers would attempt to market their programs with low fees and attractive benefits. Cost limitations would not be achieved by mandating family participation in long-term care. Cost control would be realized by making benefits available only to those with serious disabilities. Further, programs would be designed to allocate resources directly to the impaired elderly and their families and minimize administrative intervention.

## NOTES

1. Alan Sager, "Learning the Home Care Needs of the Elderly: Patient, Family and Professional Views of an Alternative to Institutionalization," mimeographed (Waltham, Mass.: Levinson Policy Institute, Heller School, 1979).

2. Francis G. Caro and Robert Morris, "Personal Care for the Severely Disabled: Organizing and Financing Care," mimeographed (Waltham, Mass.: Levinson Gerontological Policy Institute, Heller School, 1971), and Francis G. Caro, "Expanding Options for the Personal Care of the Disabled Elderly," mimeographed (Waltham, Mass.: Levinson Gerontological Policy Institute, Heller School, 1971).

3. "Second Annual Report," mimeographed (Milwaukee, Wis.: Community Care Organization of Milwaukee County, 1979).

4. Triage, "Final Report, 1979," mimeographed (Plainville, Conn.: Triage Coordinate Delivery of Service to the Elderly, 1979). As a Medicare intermediary, Triage incurred administrative costs beyond those associated with just home care. Therefore an exact figure for administrative costs is difficult to compute.

5. States are moving toward vendorizing and a Title XX administrative model for home care. It is not clear whether the strategy solves the state's management problems or simply makes them less visible. If states relinquish to vendors their authority to test disability and determine eligibility, then conflicts of interest and slippage of the states' regulatory power would seem to be inevitable. Division of functions in the maintenance model would pemit either federal or state governments to maintain control of access to benefit dollars even if they are not involved in direct management.

# Use of the Tax System
# in Home Care:
# A Brief Note

Robert Perlman

Certain families providing care for disabled relatives have, for almost 30 years, received public support through income tax deductions and lately through tax credits. It is worth reviewing this experience, not only to assess the experience with the use of the tax system for this purpose, but for the light it sheds on evolving social policy in this area.

The deduction of expenses for the care of a "disabled dependent or spouse" was adopted in 1954 along with deductions for the care of children. The primary purpose of both was to enable family members to be gainfully employed; the relief of hardship was apparently a secondary objective (Goode, 1976, pp. 155-156). Limits were placed on the amount that could be deducted per month and the deduction was phased out for families with an adjusted gross income above a certain level (Committee on the Budget, U.S. Senate, 1976, pp. 95-96).

Several new justifications beyond facilitating employment were added in 1971: (1) encouraging the hiring of domestic workers, (2) encouraging the care of incapacitated persons at home rather than in institutions, (3) providing relief to middle income as well as low income taxpayers, and (4) providing relief for employment-related expenses of household services as well as for dependent care (*op. cit.*, p. 96). In 1975 a tax credit of 20 percent was substituted for the deduction.

Payments for services provided by a dependent of the taxpayer did not qualify, thus barring the tax credit for services performed by a relative inside the home. As a result of a change in 1978, payments to *nondependent* relatives could qualify if they worked *inside* the home as well as payments to *nondependent grandparents* providing care *outside* the home.

Unfortunately, from the point of view of studying home care, child care and care of the disabled have been lumped together from the outset; this makes it very difficult to isolate and analyze the data on dependent care. Moreover, virtually all of the commentary on this provision of the tax laws has concentrated on child care (see sources at the end of this note). However, this excerpt from a private communication from the Office of Tax Analysis in the Office of the Secretary of the Treasury indicates that this provision was not seriously intended, nor was it actually used to any substantial extent, to assist families with the expense of caring for a disabled relative.

> In making estimates of the cost of revisions or proposed revisions of the child and dependent care provisions the case of disabled dependents was largely ignored. As long as the provision was an itemized deduction it was assumed that the cost of care of disabled dependents would normally be taken under the medical expense deduction provided by Section 213 of the Internal Revenue Code, since it provides no limits as the amount deductible, size of adjusted gross income, or the need for both spouses to work. As a tax credit it is now available to persons who use the standard deduction. However, even with recent liberalizations, the standard deduction is used primarily by single persons and by families of modest means, and it seems likely that most severely disabled adults in such families are taken care of through publicly financed programs such as medicaid and medicare outside the family.

Nevertheless, the Office of Tax Analysis provides a method for making an approximation of the magnitude and distribution of tax claims on behalf of families caring for a disabled member. They suggest that 10 percent of the expenses claimed and 10 percent of the cost of the tax credit be attributed to home care and 90 percent to child care (letters to the writer dated August 20, 1980 and July 14, 1978). On this basis one can estimate the number of families claiming deductions, the amount of the expenses, and the revenue loss.

First, there was a steady increase in the 1970s in the number of families using this tax provision, rising from approximately 100,000 before 1971 to 300,000 in 1978. The aggregate expense claimed for care of disabled relatives rose from $125 million in

1973 to $263 million in 1977. The tax revenue loss increased from $18 million before 1971 (Surrey, p. 201) to $66 million in 1978. The average amount of expenses claimed seems to have varied between $700 and $1400.

In describing the distribution of the tax credits in terms of family income, it is impossible to disaggregate the care of the disabled from the cost of child care. Together, claims were distributed as indicated in Table 1.

Using the data presented in this brief review, it is possible to make several observations.

1. While the number of families making use of this tax relief has increased, it still represents only a very minor part of the "family home care system" in the United States. The 300,000 families who made claims in 1978 constitute under 10 percent of all the families involved in home care.

2. From what is known about the out-of-pocket expenses of home care, the expenses submitted (ranging from $700 to $1400 on the average) seem low. To a considerable extent, this may be due to the narrow limits placed on payments to service-providers who happen—as in the case of teenagers—to be dependents of the taxpayer. If one were to calculate the dollar value of unpaid family

Table 1

Number of Returns and Amount of Tax Credit
for Child Care and Dependent Care by Family Income, 1977*

| Adjusted Gross Income | No. of Returns | Percent | Amount (in thousands) | Percent |
|---|---|---|---|---|
| Under $5,000 | 5,191 | 0.2 | $ 665 | 0.5 |
| $5,000 under $10,000 | 324,555 | 11.3 | 52,175 | 10.0 |
| $10,000 under $15,000 | 564,655 | 19.6 | 91,338 | 17.5 |
| $15,000 under $20,000 | 657,958 | 22.9 | 105,426 | 20.2 |
| $20,000 under $30,000 | 979,437 | 34.1 | 186,793 | 35.7 |
| $30,000 under $50,000 | 301,521 | 10.5 | 71,113 | 13.6 |
| $50,000 or more | 41,568 | 1.4 | 13,765 | 2.5 |
|  | 2,874,885 | 100.0 | $521,275 | 100.0 |

*All returns.

Source: Internal Revenue Service, Statistics Division, May 1978.

care, the amounts claimed under the tax law would appear almost miniscule.

3. Above all, as the Senate Committee's report and Surrey point out, this tax advantage is skewed so that it favors higher income families. In many instances it is simply not accessible to poor families, since it is available to married persons employed on a substantially full-time basis and to single persons to enable them to be gainfully employed. Poor people who are retired, or who are not working, or who are not aware of the provision, cannot benefit.

To summarize, experience to date with the tax system as a means of helping families sustain the provision of home care seems to be woefully inadequate in terms of reaching the population involved. Second, the present provisions take account of only a small part of the family's actual effort, since it excludes certain relatives' paid work and all unpaid work by family members. Third, it is seriously inequitable in terms of family income, discriminating in practice against the poor. Finally, as Surrey observes, it seems not to be the appropriate instrument for meeting the problem addressed in this book. He writes that while "tax expenditure items of this character evidence the sensitivity of the tax system to concern over the lack of federal assistance in social areas [and while] . . . Relief through the tax system is thus the point where social advance wedges into the federal budget and is often the forerunner of larger and more adequate direct programs in later years . . . Unfortunately, the tax expenditure item usually remains as an inequitable and vestigial program" (Surrey, *op. cit.,* p. 201).

## SOURCES

Committee on the Budget, U.S. Senate, *Tax Expenditure,* 94th Congress, 2nd Session, 1976.
Richard Goode, *The Individual Income Tax,* Washington, D.C.: The Brookings Institution, 1976.
Stanley S. Surrey, *Pathways to Tax Reform: The Concept of Tax Expenditures,* Cambridge, Mass.: Harvard University Press, 1973.

# Concluding Observations

Where have we arrived in this examination of family home care? What are the main issues, reasonable assumptions, and promising directions in which to move?

It seems clear that the provision of care by family members to dependent persons in their own homes is already a widespread undertaking in the United States and that it represents a growing social need. The largest group of beneficiaries of home care, the elderly, is increasing dramatically in number and in the severity of their dependence on others. There seems no reason to expect a decline in the number or proportion of children and of people in their middle years who will also require assistance with the daily tasks of living. Demand for non-professional care, in other words, shows every sign of expanding in the next quarter-century.

The care-giving families constitute a vast resource; Moroney calls it a "social service" of prime significance. Thus far, there has been no significant diminution of family care, but it is a fragile system at both the household level and the macro level, subject to threats primarily from two sources. One is a decline in the available pool of persons ready, willing, and able to fill the caring role, a decline attributable to shifts in life-styles, family composition, the distribution of sex-related activities, and people's notions of what is right and permissible in family relationships.

The second threat to the system lies in what the literature refers to as "family burden." Many, many families are overextended and are not receiving the help they need. The informal system is at risk because of the inadequacies of the very programs that potentially could sustain it. Present policies and programs tend to tilt the system away from family care and toward costly and often unnecessary institutional care, especially in nursing homes for the elderly.

Would assistance to families strengthen them by reducing their burdens or would it weaken their will and encourage them to shrug off their responsibilities to the Welfare State? Moroney found that supportive services did not reduce the volume of family-provided help for the dependent population; on the contrary, this assistance bolstered the morale of families and their willingness and ability to give care (Moroney, 1976).

There are reservations about loading too much responsibility on either family or State. Monk, in his paper in this collection, cautions against expecting too much from families and calls attention to limits imposed by trends such as the greater longevity of the elderly and their deepening dependence on their middle-age and aging children and the decline in family care-providers as a result of increased geographic separation. He suggests housing and caring arrangements as realistic alternatives to "euphoric expectations about primary support networks." But dependent persons and their families, Morris argues, ought to be wary of the ministrations of a bureaucratized Welfare State. Doubts seem to be increasing as to whether the intervention of government and of professionals is, in the end, more protective of the citizenry or more abusive of their rights and more bungling than efficient in its implementation of programs.

On balance, however, the conclusion that emerges from the discussion in these papers is that *home care should be nurtured and supported by sharing the responsibility between the State and the family*. No one has developed a comprehensive or detailed proposal for a system of supports that would be adequate to the task. Such a system, however, ought to encompass at least these main elements:

1. Bringing professional services into the home as needed (medical, nursing, physical therapy, counseling etc.).
2. Providing paraprofessional aide for physical care, companionship, home-making chores, etc. on a flexible time schedule to supplement or when necessary substitute for the family's services.
3. Compensating families for out-of-pocket expenses and (though this is debatable) for their time.
4. Providing access to institutional settings for brief respites or for more extended stays necessitated by changes in the condition of the dependent individual or in the capabilities of the family.

Attempts to move policy in the direction suggested above are very likely to encounter problems in the following areas: (a) the *cost* of such a program, (b) *political support* for it; (c) the *criteria for allocating resources* among the growing number of potential claimants, and (d) the *form in which the supportive aid* should be organized and delivered.

*Costs*: Lacking a well-developed proposal for a program along the lines outlined above, we also lack even broad estimates of the costs. There is now much discussion of the costs of long term care and increasingly there are research efforts to compare the costs of home care and institutional care (Anderson et al., 1980; Callahan, 1981; HCFA, 1981). But the researchers encounter formidable obstacles; there are wide variations not only between the two types of care, but *within* each type in terms of the physical and mental condition of the dependent person; the kind and amount of services rendered; and the costs that should be imputed for unpaid, informal services. A study in Minnesota reached these conclusions based on a comparison of a home care population and a nursing home population (Anderson et al. 1980, pp. iv and v):

> 1. Nursing home residents receive so much more of each formal service than do home care clients, that even with lower per unit costs, the average monthly cost of each formal (paid) service is substantially higher in nursing homes.

> 2. If the implicit costs of informal services are included in the cost of care, then for those home care clients who receive informal care, the average cost of nursing and personal care are higher for home care than they are for nursing home residents.

> 3. Even after controlling for differences in client characteristics, the cost of serving the nursing home sample is still significantly higher than for the home care sample. This includes only formal costs.

> 4. The amount it will cost to provide formal care to an expanded home care population will be very sensitive to both the functional disabilities of the recipients and the amount of informal care that will be provided.

The comparison between home care and institutional care was brought dramatically to the public's attention late in 1981 when television and newspapers carried the account of Katie Beckett, a 3-year-old girl in Iowa who had been in a hospital with viral encephalitis since she was four months old. President Reagan, referring to Katie in a press conference, said it was costing $6,000 a month to keep her in the hospital and that she would be better off at home and where it would cost only $1,000 a month. But if she went home her parents would lose Medicaid payments and since they could not afford to pay $1,000 a month, she remained in the hospital in yet another instance of Catch 22 regulations.

It turned out that the President had underestimated by 50 percent the cost of Katie's in-hospital and at-home care, which amounted to $12,000 and $2,500 a month respectively. But the point was clear to all: Medicaid regulations were preventing the family from having their child at home and were, on top of that, costing society almost $10,000 in avoidable expenses.

The findings of the Minnesota study quoted above reinforce what has been said many times in these pages. A substantial reduction of home care and the consequent transfer of people to institutional settings would bring a further rise in costs that have already skyrocketed. The cost of nursing home services rose from $800 million in 1967 to $6.4 billion in 1977 (Callahan et al., 1979, p. 7). Expenditures for long-term care, according to estimates by the Congressional Budget Office, will amount to $64-$75 billion by the mid-1980s (Morris and Youket, 1980, p. 8).

Expenditures of these magnitudes give an indication of what might be the financial result of a decline in family home care, which now provides more than three times the amount of care rendered by formal sources. However, the figures do not shed much light on the costs that a truly adequate system of supports for these families would add to current or projected expenditures. In his paper, Farber expresses some concern about the infinite nature of "need," the great growth of the helping industry, and the possibilities of fraud. On the other hand, Sager found that decisions about the kind and level of care that were made by elderly people and their families were by no means unrealistic or unjustified and that "fears of uncontrollable spending ensuing from patient or family influence over care planning find no support" in his study.

*Political support*: How much more this society is willing to give to families to sustain the care they provide to dependent individuals is, clearly, a political issue. We pointed out in the Introduction to Part I that the question arises at a juncture in the evolution of social policy in this country, when opponents of the Welfare State are seeking to reverse the growth of social programs, a process that began in the Carter Administration and is continuing, at a much accelerated tempo, in the Reagan Administration.

Research on popular support for a program such as that projected here has not been undertaken. One researcher suggests that there is a reservoir of support in the United States for assistance to the disabled, especially the elderly disabled (Cook, 1979). It is not unreasonable to think that political support for a program of home care would tap into the positive feelings Americans have about conditions that are "beyond the control" or responsibility of the individual affected (Coughlin, 1980).

Such questions, however, are never dealt with in the abstract, particularly in legislative bodies. They are confronted as choices among competing programs and constituencies. In that light and in a period of drastic budget-cutting, it is not easy to be sanguine about larger appropriations for assisting families who provide home care, though it remains to be seen to what extent the elderly will press politically for.this in the years ahead.

*Criteria for allocating resources*: The aggregate costs of an adequate program for supporting family care and the political support it may enjoy will be closely related to the bases on which assistance is given. A program that is limited by tight eligibility regulations in terms of family income or the physical condition of the dependent person will obviously cost less than a broad, universal program accessible to families regardless of income and with a liberal interpretation of need for assistance. In view of the costs that can accrue to a particular family—both the direct financial outlays and the non-monetary costs that have been described in these pages—there might be some political backing for a non-means tested program. The present climate of cutbacks in social programs, however, can be expected to set rather narrow limits on the growth of expenditures in this area.

Questions of equity must also be considered. Very little, however, is known about the distribution of care-providing families in terms of their geographic location, their incomes, or the degree of dependence and the specific disabilities of their dependent relatives. For example, the geographic distribution of these families needs to be studied in relation to the availability of services. How well are the two matched in rural as distinct from urban areas and from state to state? One nationwide search to uncover projects designed to help families care for a disabled relative located only a few such projects in 11 states. This raises a question as to whether these special efforts, as well as basic services such as homemaker and home health aide programs, are appropriately distributed across the country (Zimmerman, 1979).

The discriminatory effects of income-eligibility policies on family care have been stressed so much that they require little elaboration here. Those who are eligible for Medicaid, Title XX, Veterans Administration, and other benefits receive some assistance. Many families not eligible because of an income "surplus" are struggling under heavy financial and other burdens. This problem merits study to learn how much of an increase in the income limits in these programs would help how many families, how much, and at what cost.

We have seen evidence that the present structure of benefits discriminates against certain families in terms of the specific circumstances or disability of their dependent relative. This was the case with schizophrenics, as shown by Hart in her paper. Morell argues that within the retarded population, children living at home are shortchanged by the higher priority that is given to adults living in the community. Morris comments that the more severe kinds of dependencies are avoided by service providers who "cream" off the less demanding, less repugnant kinds of situations and bypass the more difficult ones. There are simply illustrations of the inequities that need investigation in order to arrive at sound policies governing distribution of benefits.

*The form that assistance should take*: Should there be cash assistance or the provision of services? There are experiments with these two methods, but it is too early to report definitive results (Zimmerman, 1979, pp. 88-89). Should insurance coverage, public or private, be utilized to protect families from home care as an insurable risk? Should the tax system be used?

To these questions one must add the query: to whom should benefits, whether in cash or in kind, be channeled: to the dependent person or the family? This becomes, in effect, a matter of legal rights in which self-determination for the individual must be balanced against problems of mental competence and against the rights of the other family members.

The notion of providing material incentives to families has been argued pro and con. Callahan considers it prudent "to develop policies that will reinforce incentives to families so that choices other than institutional care will be available," a strategy he favors to "avoid the legal, political, and administrative traps that lie in the path of uncertain deterrent approaches" (Callahan et al. 1979, pp. iv-v). The incentives he suggests include more financial and non-financial aid to families, as well as tax credits and insurance programs. Prager, on the other hand, found many reasons to oppose a 1975 Senate bill that would have given financial subsidies to families caring for an elderly dependent. Among his objections he stated that "the resultant exchange relationship must demean the value of the service given by the family" (Prager, 1977, p. 60).

The weight of the evidence in the foregoing papers favors Callahan's position and challenges the premises that underlie Prager's argument. However, experience with tax credits, which are included in Callahan's list of possibilities, is not reassuring. In the brief account, above, of this experience, it seems to have operated with a built-in bias toward higher income families and discriminated against the poor.

It must be apparent at this stage that the issues of cost, of political appeal, of the criteria for providing aid and the forms it should take are all thoroughly interlocked. It is beyond the scope of this work to set forth in detail the programmatic specifications for coping with these issues. Such a proposal will require more information and more debate. There is much that is not known about the extent and nature of family home care in this country. Hopefully, for both humane and economic reasons, further study will be supported. There is more public discussion of the problem and that can only be welcomed by the dependent people we have discussed and by their families, and by the rest of us who, for the moment at least, are in neither of those categories.

# References to Introductory Sections

Acford, Joanne P. "Reducing Medicaid Expenditures Through Family Responsibility: Critique of a Recent Proposal," *Law and Medicine* May 1979.

Aldrich, Robert et al. *The Mental Retardation Service Delivery Project,* Olympic, Wa.: Washington State Department of Social and Health Services, 1971.

Allan, Kathryn H. "First Findings of the 1972 Survey of the Disabled: General Characteristics." *Social Security Bulletin* 39, October 1976: 18-37.

Allan, Kathryn H. and Mildred E. Cinsky. "General Characteristics of the Disabled Population," *Social Security Survey of the Disabled, 1966,* Report No. 19 DHEW Publication No. (SSA) 72-11713. Washington, D.C.: U.S. Department of Health, Education, and Welfare, Social Security Administration, Office of Research and Statistics, July 1972.

Anderson, Nancy N., Sharon Patten, and Jay N. Greenberg. *A Comparison of Home Care and Nursing Home Care for Older Persons in Minnesota, Vol. III–Summary.* University of Minnesota, 1980.

Barry, Patricia, "Summary of the Comprehensive Needs Study," The Urban Institute (Working Paper 0981-04), 1975.

Bennett, Ruth, David Wilder, Jeanne Teresi. *Personal Time Dependency and Family Attitudes.* New York: Community Council of Greater New York, 1978.

Berkowitz, Monroe, William G. Johnson and Edward H. Murphy. PUBLIC POLICY TOWARD DISABILITY. New York: Prager Publishers, 1976.

Boggs, Elizabeth M. and R. Lee Henney. *A Numerical and Functional Description of the Developmentally Disabled Population in the United States by Major Life Activities as Defined in the Developmental Disabilities Assistance and Bill of Rights Act as amended in PL 95-602,* unpublished paper, EMC Institute, Philadelphia.

Bradshaw, J. and D. Lawton, "Tracing the Causes of Stress in Families with Handicapped Children," *British Journal of Social Work,* 8:2, pp. 181-191, 1978.

Branch, Laurence G. and Floyd J. Fowler, Jr. *The Health Care Needs of the Elderly and Chronically Disabled in Massachusetts.* Boston: University of Massachusetts Survey Research Program, March 1975.

Brownstein, Elise and Helen G. Berkley. "Medical Social Work Home Intervention Project." Boston: The Children's Hospital Medical Center, 1979, unpublished.

Bruininks, Robert H. "The Needs of Families" in R.H. Bruininks and Gordon C. Krantz, *Family Care of Developmentally Disabled Members: Conference Proceedings,* University of Minnesota, 1979.

Callahan, James J., Jr., Lawrence D. Diamond, Janet Z. Giele, and Robert Morris. "Responsibility of Families for Their Severely Disabled Elders," Center for Health Policy Analysis and Research, Brandeis University, 1979.

Callahan, James J., Jr., Alonzo L. Plough, and Steve Wisensale, *Long-Term Care of Children,* University Health Policy Consortium, Brandeis University, 1981.

Callahan, James J., Jr., and Stanley S. Wallack. *Reforming the Long-Term Care System,* Lexington, Mass.: Lexington Books, 1981.

Comptroller General of the United States, *Report to Congress,* "Home Health—The Need for a National Policy to Better Provide for the Elderly." Washington, D.C.: General Accounting Office, 1977.

Cook, Fay Lomax. *Who Should Be Helped? Public Support for Social Services.* Beverly Hills, California: Sage Publications, 1979.

Coughlin, Richard M., *Ideology, Public Opinion and Welfare Policy: Attitudes Toward Taxes and Spending in Industrialized Societies*, Berkeley: University of California Press, 1980.

Danis, Benjamin C. "Stress in Individual Caring for Ill Elderly Relatives," Paper presented at the Annual Meeting of the Gerontological Society, Dallas, Texas, 1978.

DeJong, Gerben. "The Need for Personal Care Services by Severely Physically Disabled Citizens of Massachusetts." Levinson Policy Institute, Brandeis University, 1977.

Dunlap, W.R. and J.S. Hollingsworth, "How Does a Handicapped Child Affect the Family: Implications for Practitioners," *The Family Coordinator,* July 1977. (Quoted in Bruininks and Krantz, 1979.)

ELIZABETH (43) 1, Ch. 2, Sec. 7 (1601), Elizabethan Poor Laws.

Farber, Bernard. "Effects of a Severely Mentally Retarded Child on Family Integration," *Monographs of the Society for Research in Child Development,* 1959. Vol. 24, No. 2.

Fein, Joshua. "Away From Home: A Study of Deinstitutionalization and the Family of the Mentally Retarded Person," unpublished paper, Waltham, Mass.: Brandeis University, 1978.

Fotheringham, John B., Mora Skelton, and Bernard A. Hoddinott. "The Retarded Child and His Family: The Effects of Home and Institution." Ontario: The Ontario Institute for Studies in Education, 1971.

Frankfather, Dwight L., Michael J. Smith and Francis G. Caro, *Family Care of the Elderly: Public Initiatives and Private Obligations,* Lexington: Lexington Books, 1981.

Franklin, Paula A. "Impact of Disability on the Family Structure." Social Security Bulletin, Vol. 1, No. 40, May 1977.

Gaylin, Willard. "In the Beginning: Helpless and Dependent," in *Doing Good: The Limits of Benevolence,* Willard Gaylin, Ira Glasser, Steven Marcus, and David J. Rothman. New York: Pantheon Books, 1978.

Giele, Janet Z. "A Review of Selected Data Sources on the Family's Role in Long-Term Care," unpublished working paper, Levinson Policy Institute, Brandeis University, June 1980.

Glendon, Mary Ann. *The New Family and the New Property.* Woburn, MA.: Butterworths, 1981.

Gordon, Elizabeth. *Living with a Handicapped Child: A Literature Review,* Jerusalem: Ministry of Labor and Social Affairs, 1980.

Gurland, Barry, Laura Dean, Diana Cook, Roni Gurland. *Personal Time Dependency in the Elderly of New York City: Findings from the U.S.-U.K. Cross-National Geriatric Community Study.* New York: Community Council of Greater New York, 1978.

Health Care Financing Administration. *Long Term Care: Background and Future Directions,* Washington, D.C., 1981.

Howell, S.E. "Psychiatric Aspects of Rehabilitation," *Pediatric Clinics of North America,* 1973, 20, 203.

Johnson, William. "Caring for the Vulnerable Family Member: The Moral Issues," unpublished paper, Brandeis University, 1978.

Kahn, Alfred J. and Sheila Kamerman. *Not For the Poor Alone: European Social Services.* Philadelphia: Temple University Press, 1975.

Kew, Stephen. *Handicap and Family Crisis: A Study of the Siblings of Handicapped Children.* London: Pitman, 1975.

Krause, Harry D. *Family Law in a Nutshell.* St. Paul, Minn.: West Publishing Company, 1977, p. 180.

Krauss, Marty W. and Ann E. MacEachorn. "National Study of Social Services to Handicapped Children and Their Families." Report to U.S. Children's Bureau, Administration for Children Youth, and Families." Waltham, MA.: Brandeis University, 1981.

Lopes, James L. "Filial Support and Family Solidarity," 6 *Pacific Law Journal* 508, 1975.

Maddox, G. "Families as Context and Resource in Chronic Illness," in Sylvia Sherwood, ed., *Long-Term Care.* New York: Spectrum, 1975.

Maybanks, Sheila and Marvin Bryce. *Home-Based Services for Children and Families: Policy, Practice, and Research*. Springfield, Ill.: Charles C. Thomas Publishers, 1979.

Moroney, Robert M. *The Family and the State: Considerations for Social Policy*. New York: Longmans, 1976.

Moroney, Robert M. *Families, Social Services, and Social Policy: The Issue of Shared Responsibility*. U.S. Department of Health and Human Services, Public Health Service, Washington, D.C., 1980.

Morris, Robert and Paul Youket. "Major Options in Long-Term Care—Background and Framework," in Stanley S. Wallack and James J. Callahan, Jr. *Major Reforms in Long-Term Care: A Systematic Comparison of the Options*. Center for Health Policy Analysis and Research, Brandeis University, 1980.

Nagi, Saad A. "An Epidemiology of Disability Among Adults in the United States." Columbus, Ohio: Mershon Center, Ohio State University, mimeo. 1975.

National Center for Health Statistics. *Limitation of Activity and Mobility Due to Chronic Conditions, United States, 1972;* Vital and Health Statistics, Series 10 No. 96; DHEW Publication No. (HRS) 75-1523. Washington, D.C.: U.S. Department of Health, Education, and Welfare, November 1974.

Perlman, Robert and Janet Z. Giele. "Family Home Care of the Elderly." Waltham, MA.: Brandeis University, research proposal, 1979.

Perlman, Robert and Roland L. Warren. *Families in the Energy Crisis: Impacts and Implications for Theory and Policy*. Cambridge, MA.: Ballinger Publishing Company, 1977.

Prager, Edward. "On Incentives for Family Care of Aged Kin: An Exchange Theory Perspective." *The Journal of Applied Social Sciences,* January 1977, Case Western Reserve University.

Project Share. *Home Care Services*. Human Services Bibliography Series, Rockville, MD., July 1981.

Rosenbaum, Michael. "Are Family Responsibility Laws Constitutional?" 1 *Family Law Quarterly,* 55, 66 December 1967.

Schorr, Alvin. ". . . 'Thy Father and Thy Mother' . . . A Second Look at Filial Responsibility and Family Policy." Washington, D.C.: Social Security Administration, Office of Policy, Office of Research and Statistics, 1980.

Skarnulis, Edward. "Support, Not Supplant, the Natural Home: Serving Handicapped Children and Adults" in Sheila Maybanks and Marvin Bryce, *Home-Based Services for Children and Families: Policy, Practice, and Research*. Springfield, Ill.: Charles C. Thomas Publishers, 1979, p. 69.

U.S. Bureau of the Census. *General Social and Economic Characteristics: Massachusetts*. 1970 Census of Population, PC(1)-C23. Washington, D.C.: U.S. Department of Commerce, Social and Economics Statistics Administration, Bureau of the Census, April 1972.

U.S. Bureau of the Census. *Persons With Disability*, 1970 Census of Population, PC(2)-6C. Washington, D.C.: U.S. Department of Commerce, Social and Economics Administration, Bureau of the Census, January 1973a.

U.S. Bureau of the Census. *Characteristics of the Population: Massachusetts,* 1970 Census of Population, Vol. 1, Part 23. Washington, D.C.: U.S. Department of Commerce, Social and Economics Administration, Bureau of the Census, February 1973b.

U.S. Bureau of the Census. *Characteristics of the Population: United States Summary*; Vol. 1, Part 1, Section 1: 1970 Census of Population. Washington, D.C.: U.S. Department of Commerce, Social and Economics Administration, Bureau of the Census, June 1973c.

U.S. Bureau of the Census, Current Population Reports, Series P-60, No. 110, "Money Income and Poverty Status in 1975 of Families and Persons in the United States and the Northeast Region, by Divisions and States (Spring 1976 Survey of Income and Education)," U.S. Government Printing Office, Washington, D.C., 1978.

U.S. Department of Health, Education, and Welfare. Office of the Secretary. "Memorandum for July 14, 1978 Briefing, Major Initiative: Long-Term Care/Community Services," 1979. Appendix 2, "In-Home Services."

Wawzonek, Sally J. "The Role of the Family in Disability." *American Archives of Rehabilitation Therapy,* Vol. 22, No. 3, September 1974.

Zimmerman, Shirley Lee. "Families of the Developmentally Disabled: Implications for Research and the Planning and Provision of Services," in Bruininks and Krantz, *Family Care of Developmentally Disabled Members: Conference Proceedings,* University of Minnesota, 1979.